FULLY ALIVE

Gloria Gage

1 John 4:12
Gloria Gage

ACCENT BOOKS
Denver, Colorado

ACCENT BOOKS
A division of Accent Publications, Inc.
12100 W. Sixth Avenue
P.O. Box 15337
Denver, Colorado 80215

Printed in the United States of America

Library of Congress Catalog Card Number: 80-68884

ISBN 0-89636-064-4

Introduction

Fully Alive! is a result of contributions made by many people, but mostly by Wendy Dean Hickman himself, through his letters, and the events and conversations remembered by those who've loved him. It has been compiled after numerous interviews with family, teachers, classmates, coaches, teammates, and dear friends.

While the events in the story actually happened, a few of the characters have been combined to provide for both their individual privacy and smoother readability.

It is, however, an incomplete story, because, even as you are reading it, the special legacy of love and faith which Wendy gave to this world is continuing to grow and blossom in countless ways.

There are some who were introduced to Christ through Wendy's testimony and example. There are many whose lives will be forever richer for having known him.

This summer of 1981 a 450-acre Christian Retreat will open its gates in the beautiful Pine Woods of East Texas. Above the entrance, the sign reads "WENDY'S MEADOW." Brought together over the last several years by the efforts of Wendy's parents, friends, and others, it will remain as a living tribute, allowing hundreds of young people and adults an opportunity to share in the wonders of God's world and to become refreshed as they fellowship with each other and with nature.

A fitting tribute for Wendy Dean Hickman—who saw God's handiwork in a highway of stars in a summer night sky, and felt the rebirth of Christ's love in the first spring blossoms of hyacinths.

He believed that Christ is man's only "stepping-stone" to God. What more meaning could his life have held, than for Wendy, himself, to be a stepping-stone guiding others to his Lord?

What more can any life offer, than to be a continuation of God's love in this world?

Gloria Gage
May, 1981

1.

It was nine o'clock. Kent could set his watch when he looked down from the upstairs window and saw him running up the drive.

Every Saturday Kent Conine could remember, his friend, Wendy, would jog the short mile from his house to Kent's, arriving at nine o'clock sharp.

But this Saturday was different.

Today—Wendy Dean Hickman would not be coming!

Kent sat before his upstairs window staring blankly out over the driveway . . .

The boys paced themselves, jogging with the smooth, easy rhythm that comes only from hours of practice. Wendy breathed deeply, relishing the sensations which pulsed through his strong young body as he forced all his energies into disciplined obedience.

Kent moved at his side with long, measured strides, like a thoroughbred eager to be granted the freedom of a loose rein. They moved together, picking up the pace on the straight-a-way, moving faster and faster, until suddenly it ceased to be a practice lap and became a two-man race, each of them making an all-out effort to win.

Nearing the end of the lap both boys stretched into full stride, pounding ahead, every muscle and fiber forced to its limit. Kent strained his long legs, inching ahead, one step, then two. As the other boys working-out on the field became aware of the drama on the track, whistles and shouts of encouragement began to build into an enthusiastic chorus.

Kent plunged across the finish first with Wendy struggling vainly to close in. They both slowed to a walk, perspiration beading up and trickling into small soaking streams on their skin.

"It's a good thing we weren't racing," Wendy gasped, his breath returning with deep, heavy gulps. "One of these days I'm going to slip past and let *you* push for a change!"

"That'll be the day!"

They both laughed good-naturedly and joined the others, already into calisthenics. Following a rigorous workout, they pulled on pads and helmets for the toughest part yet to come.

The crunch of pads slamming against each other resounded in their ears and the smell of sweat invaded their nostrils. Still they plunged ahead, clashing to the rhythmic cadence of the coach's voice until at last his shrill whistle sounded a reprieve.

"Okay, you guys, hit the showers, and tomorrow I want to see a little muscle out here!"

Kent's legs felt like two-hundred-pound weights as he dragged himself to the locker room, already steamed and noisy. He collapsed on the bench and wondered if he'd recover enough to take off his gear, or if his arms might fall off when he tried.

He lifted his head slowly to be sure it was still attached and looked straight up into a friendly, smiling face.

Wendy didn't say a word, just grinned, turned around and taped a small piece of paper on the inside door of Kent's locker and walked off toward the showers. It wasn't long before curiosity outweighed Kent's weariness and he got up to look. In neatly printed letters, Wendy had written, "Smile, Kent, God loves you!"

Kent did smile, in spite of himself. Then, just as a way of saying thank you, he hid all Wendy's clothes in the broom closet.

Wendy and Kent had been friends since junior high school, when they first faced each other on the football field. Kent was a natural at the quarterback position, using his strength and agility to move the ball quickly up the middle or roll out for a spiraling pass.

Wendy played defensive end, the "monster-man" position. He was lighter than Kent, but anything he lacked in size, he more than made up in that sheer determination of his.

The friendly competition between them first began in a junior high practice scrimmage. Coach Keck called a halfback option pass, but the receiver slipped and went down. Kent was left with a "busted play" and no one to take the ball. He made a fast adjustment, tucked the ball away and ran a slant toward the corner of the defensive line—right at Wendy.

Kent faked to the inside, then jumped back toward the sideline. Wendy tried to cut back with him, lost his footing and fell hard on the turf. Kent saw his opportunity, with nothing but thirty yards of open field between him and the goal line. But he hadn't figured on his opponent's tenacity.

Even as he hit the ground, Wendy didn't give up, but rolled once and stretched full out to grasp Kent's ankle as he darted down the sidelines. The ground suddenly rose up to greet him in surprise. A few minutes later, Kent staggered back to the huddle, angry at losing his chance, but with a lot more respect for a defensive end named Wendy Hickman.

Football played a very big part in both of the boys' lives. Wendy's Dad played ball in college and naturally hoped his son would follow in his footsteps. From the time he learned to walk, Wendy was playing catch with a small rubber version of the pigskin. He spent many hours romping with his Dad, and later with his brother, Andy. The two small boys would race to throw their tiny arms about their father's legs in a mock tackle and the 200-pound man would fall to the ground "helpless" against the mighty force of his eager sons.

Kent's Dad was a great armchair quarterback, encouraging his boy to shine in the sport, taking pride in his ability as an extension of his own masculine ambition.

High school football was more than a game—it was a disciplined art — powerfully able to join father and son in a bond of personal pride and closeness.

Wendy and Kent both sensed this power and learned to deal with it, each in his own way. Kent found it easy to play the casual hero, and his natural athletic ability seldom let him down. He got by with half the effort; yet, somehow, things usually seemed to go his way.

For Wendy, it wasn't quite so easy and, as a result, he learned a great deal more. He discovered that, by his own force of will, he could reach goals even beyond his physical expectations. Football presented a challenge which he was determined to master. Small defeats only served to enflame his ambition and thus the rewards for success were even more valuable.

In one-on-one confrontations, like the impromptu race that day, Kent invariably came out ahead, but Wendy proved by his response to these minor defeats that his sense of competition was more within himself than against anyone else. He believed deeply in doing all that he could with the talents he possessed. A certain fierceness about his attitude kept him continually reaching for that one second faster than yesterday, that one yard more today.

In high school, while their friendship had deepened, the competition between them was as strong as ever. Meanwhile Kent grew more and more aware that Wendy's strength came not just from his own will, but from a spiritual source. It wasn't something he flaunted or pushed on anyone else, but it was always there, like a deep well that never lacked, as a source of faith and purpose.

Kent longed for the same faith and peace his friend possessed, but somehow it eluded him. "It works for *you,* Wendy," he once admitted, "but I have to count on myself. I believe God gave me strength to stand on my own and follow my own instincts."

"I know, Kent. But, unless you depend on Him to guide you, your instincts can get pretty lonely. Someday you're going to find you can't handle it alone. And then you'll know what it is to let go completely, and put everything in His hands and trust Him completely."

It was impossible for Kent to admit his doubts, even to himself. Habit had taught him to keep all areas of vulnerability buried beneath a confident, fun-loving exterior. Admitting any weakness might create a chink in the protective armor he had succeeded in building around himself. He could accept God's love for man as His creation, but to confess a need for help on a personal level from a personal Saviour meant relinquishing control, and that was something he couldn't allow.

A brisk shower after the tough practice revived his tired muscles and a hint of warmth in the air restored his spirit. Kent suddenly felt too good to think about negative possibilities. It was spring! He could taste it like fresh strawberries floating on the air as he and Wendy walked toward their cars. Honeysuckle vines along the fence were stirring to life with promises of sweetness to come, and grasshoppers were just beginning their practice leaps over new green sprouts.

"Everything is so alive this time of year," Kent said, thinking out loud. "Even the old split tree is putting out new leaves."

Wendy nodded in agreement as they passed an old oak tree ravaged long ago by some harsh winter's storm.

They walked side by side in silence, each renewing his own private acquaintance with the approaching season.

The boys soon reached the parking lot and Wendy's pickup truck. There Wendy paused, shifting his books and the heavy athletic bag onto one arm while he dug into his pocket for his keys. He leaned heavily against the truck for a minute. "You know, Kent, I think I'd like to be a science teacher. Mr. Zidermanis makes it so interesting. He's been talking about life cycles and the balance of nature."

Kent couldn't help smiling as he glanced at the familiar faraway look in his friend's hazel eyes as he talked. He knew Wendy's ambitions far exceeded his own. Wendy wanted to *see everything* and *do everything*. Kent had a lot of interests too, but no definite ideas about the future—not yet anyway. Wendy was fascinated by antique cars, he yearned to travel, to study science and biology, maybe even archaeology. He already knew more of the Bible than Kent had even read, and now, he was talking about becoming, of all things, a school teacher!

"Who knows," Wendy was saying, "maybe some day . . ."

"Hey!" voices interrupted from behind them. "How 'bout a lift home?"

Their deep thoughts were abruptly dismissed as they were joined by a gang of friends. And, off they went, three guys crammed in Kent's beat-up green Chevy and Wendy following right behind with two more in his pickup.

No one remembers who thought of it, but Hal was elected the culprit. When they stopped for a red light at a busy intersection, Hal jumped out, ran back to Wendy's truck, quickly opened the hood and yanked off the coil wire, killing the engine. Then, as boys were bursting from both sides of the truck, Hal jumped back into the Chevy just as the light turned green. As they sped away, Kent looked in his rear view mirror and saw Wendy bending under his hood, and a long line of cars behind him with horns blasting.

Wheels were the cause of a lot of pranks, but they were also a great asset when it came to solving the boys' biggest problem—girls! Wendy was a little shy in that direction, a quality that was itself appealing to the opposite sex, not to mention his blond hair, deep hazel eyes and beautiful manners, while Kent's dark features and abrupt sense of humor were distinctly different, but equally attractive. And since Kent was a "self-proclaimed expert" on girls, it was natural for Wendy to ask his advice on occasion.

Wendy and Amy had been dating for a few weeks. Friday was her birthday and he planned a special evening, but as usual had come to Kent for help.

"I'm going to do it," he said, "Amy will be sixteen, and she should be kissed on her birthday! But, I'm kinda worried. What'll I say? What'll I do?"

"Aw, Wendy, you've kissed girls before. What's the matter?"

"I know, I know, but Amy's different. She's . . . special."

"You don't have to *say* anything," Kent told him gently. "Just walk up, put your arms around her and kiss her! That's all there is to it. And don't worry!"

That evening as Wendy walked Amy to her door to say goodnight, his nervousness was evident. Amy's voice was soft, her fingers touching the gold chain on her throat. "Thanks again for the necklace. I love it . . . . It was a very special birthday for me."

Without even thinking, Wendy heard himself saying, "Amy, would you mind if we prayed together?"

Startled, Amy hesitated a moment. It was certainly the last thing she had expected him to ask. "Of course not," she murmured at last.

He took her hand and spoke quietly, his voice so natural and sincere, she felt genuinely touched.

"Dear Father," Wendy prayed, "thank you for Your gifts to us; for friends, for the good times we enjoy, and for Your strength and Your love. And thank You for Amy and allowing me to share her special day. Watch over her and keep her always safe."

It seemed the most natural thing in the world to Amy for Wendy to put his arms around her and kiss her, as if they'd been saying goodnight that way for years.

It was only later in her room alone, that she realized it was their first kiss, and she smiled at herself in the mirror, thinking what a perfect birthday it had been.

Only a few weeks later, another minor crisis developed. The boys were working-out in the school gym one afternoon. Wendy lay stretched on the leg-curl, pulling his knees tightly until he could feel the strain on his calf muscles. Beads of perspiration had begun to dampen his blond hair when he paused, "You know the drill-team party next week, Kent? Amy asked me to go with her. I told her that I am kind of shy when I go to things like that, but she said that doesn't matter—that she was sure I'd have a good time. What do you think?"

"Hey, Wendy, this is the one big event of the year when the Drill Team ask the guys. So, she wouldn't have asked you if she didn't really want you to go, right?"

"Yeah, but . . ." Wendy sat up but still looked very doubtful.

"Aw, come on, bozo. We'll have a ball." Kent slugged him on the arm and bounced around like a fighter, shadow-boxing with the wall. "Maybe I can even arrange to run out of gas on the way home."

"Oh, brother!" Wendy's face turned slightly orange as he quickly turned back to his exercises. "You've got a one-track mind, Romeo!"

"Hey, that's not bad—" Kent stopped to contemplate, "The New World Middleweight Champion—Romeo the Great!"

With that, he danced around, hands clasped above his head in the traditional victory signal. So enthralled was he in his illusion, that he stepped back blindly and caught his foot on the dangling free bar weight of the Dorsi machine. The ensuing clatter took on disastrous proportions, attracting the attention of a large crowd, both faculty and students.

It was a classic picture of a true "champion," sprawled flat on his back, both arms entangled in the metal frame of the bench press and one leg suspended in midair, a foot firmly wedged in the tension cord of the leg-curl.

The brief second of stunned silence was shattered by raucous laughter. Wendy joined Kent on the floor rolling in unrestrained glee.

This time it was Kent who turned a bright shade of orange, just momentarily, before he gave in and joined the others in their merriment.

At nine Saturday morning, as usual, Wendy came running up the drive. Kent was still in bed. He heard a whistle but tried to pretend it was just some misguided bird. Finally he dragged himself to the window and stuck his head out.

"Come back in August," he yelled down.

Wendy laughed and called back, "Come on, Kent. Remember you said you'd help me put up that mailbox at Amy's. Then, we're going on a picnic."

"Okay, okay, but it's a plot to turn me into an old man and deny the world a great lover!"

He pulled on some jeans and a sweatshirt, splashed a little cold water on his face and stumbled down the stairs. There was a note on the kitchen table—

> *"Hi Nite Owl!*
>
> *I'm off to do some shopping. Don't forget it's your day to cut the lawn. See you at 6:00 for dinner.*
>
> *Love,*
> *Mom"*

"Aw! I wonder if Paul Newman ever had to cut the grass," he thought out loud as he grabbed a couple of apples and started out the door.

Wendy was waiting patiently in front, staring up at a tree limb which stretched toward the roof. "Look," he whispered, "that squirrel has found a way into your attic. He's moving in."

Sure enough, the little furry rascal was making repeated trips from a hole high in the tree's trunk carrying a pouch full of his belongings down the limb, dropping noiselessly to the roof, and disappearing under an eave.

Wendy laughed and said, "You'd better tell your dad, before he sets up housekeeping and raises a family."

"Yeah, I guess I better. He's playing golf this morning, but I'll be sure and tell him later. Here, have an apple," he said yawning.

Wendy bit off a small piece of the apple and pitched it up on the roof near the eave. As they started walking, Kent tried to shake his brain awake. "What did you say we were supposed to do today?"

"I told Amy we'd come over and set up their new mailbox," Wendy reminded him between mouthfuls of apple. "Her Dad's out of town and her Mom would really like to get it put up. It's one of those boxes on a post. We'll have to sink it in some concrete, but it shouldn't take long. And Amy and Carol are fixing lunch for a picnic at the lake. We can take the trail bikes along and do some riding. Dad already said it would be all right if we stay on the trail and take it easy with the girls. Okay?"

"Sure," Kent answered and yawned again. "What do you suppose the girls are going to fix for lunch? Say! Where are we walking to anyway?" It suddenly dawned on him that they had already walked two blocks.

"I had to think of some way to wake you up. We're just going back by my house to get the truck and load the bikes. Besides, you can use the exercise, Tubby!"

With that remark Wendy took off running. Kent charged after him, wide awake now and full of mock anger. They arrived side by side, laughing and puffing, and walked around to the back gate to get the bikes from the storeroom where they were greeted enthusiastically by "Otis," the Hickmans' Saint Bernard. Kent always accused him of being a Shetland pony in disguise. *No one,* friend or foe, walked past Otis without a wet, but invariably friendly, hello.

Within a few minutes they managed to load the trail bikes, with a lot of noisy help from Otis, and started off to Amy's.

"Hey, what's this?" Kent asked, picking up a strangelooking rock sculpture from the seat.

Wendy's cheeks turned crimson as he answered, "Oh, it's just a little something I made for Amy."

"Oh, I see. That's real cute, Wendy. And I always thought the only kind of rocks girls went for were the ones with 'karats'!"

While Kent roared with laughter, Wendy just drove on, ignoring his teasing remarks about the little figure of a football player that he had made by gluing small rocks together. It was actually quite clever and Kent was certain Amy would love it, but he never missed an opportunity to tease Wendy where girls were concerned.

It took most of the morning to dig a hole, brace the post and pour the concrete. "Boy, that lunch the girls are fixing better be somethin'. All this work is sure making me hungry," Kent groaned as they finished smoothing the wet cement around the square post.

By the time they were cleaned up, the girls were ready with the food—a big picnic basket which smelled very tempting.

The four of them, wedged tightly into the cab of the pickup, talked and laughed all the way to the lake. It was a beautiful, warm day and they were caught up with the joyous sensations of youthful spring fever.

Turning off the highway onto a side road which climbed through a densely wooded area, they came out atop a high hill, green and lush with new grass. Circling the hill just at the edge of the tree line was a well-worn trail, scarred by the tracks of countless cycle riders. Below them, the lake shimmered in the sunlight like a crystal punchbowl dotted with a hundred marshmallow sailboats.

It was an enchanting picture, but the boys spent little time enjoying it, so anxious were they to exhibit their prowess on the bikes for the girls. First, they drove one loop of the trail checking for dips or holes to be avoided. Then, the girls climbed on behind, clinging tightly to them and squealing at every bump and curve of the path.

As they sped along the trail high above the lake, Wendy felt deliriously happy. As Amy giggled in delight and held her arms more tightly around him, he was filled with the simple pleasures of her closeness and the beauty of the world whirling around them. For a brief moment, they were a part of nature and felt as if they had been lifted from the earth to sail free.

At last, breathless and windblown, the boys delivered their passengers back to the truck.

"That was some ride!" Amy gasped.

"I didn't scare you, did I? Did I go too fast?" Wendy asked.

"Oh, no! I loved it. And I felt perfectly safe with you."

"Well, I'm not too sure about myself," Carol exclaimed. "I think Kent was trying to deliberately rearrange my anatomy!"

"I wouldn't do that! I kinda like it just the way it is," Kent teased.

Grabbing the picnic basket from the back of the truck, he raced up the hill with Carol right behind him, threatening him at every step if he should spill their carefully packed lunch.

Wendy took Amy's hand and together they started up the gentle slope, totally oblivious to the inane chatterings coming from above them.

Carol spread a blanket under the trees and Amy took a red checkered cloth from the basket and opened it out on the ground beside them.

"Here, make yourself useful. Think you can handle opening these?" Carol chided, handing Kent a 6-pak of Cokes.

Kent reached out for the drinks, then suddenly collapsed to the ground holding his stomach and gasping, "I'm too weak. Feed me quick before I faint!"

"Oh, you nut!" Carol laughed and gave him a shove which started him rolling down the hill.

The girls just ignored him and went on unpacking fried chicken, potato chips, pickles and chocolate cupcakes.

Wearing a dubious frown, Wendy picked up a chicken leg and asked, "This wouldn't, by any chance, be one of those Easter chickens, would it, Amy?"

Amy turned with a shocked expression on her face. "Oh, Wendy, of course not! And it isn't Easter Rabbit either!"

Both of them burst out laughing. Finally they composed themselves enough to explain the joke to the others.

"You remember, Kent," Wendy began, "when Amy came over to my house early on Easter morning and decorated the whole front yard with notes leading me from one place to another like a treasure hunt. I looked under every shrub and rock and behind every tree for half an hour. Finally, behind a huge bush on the side of the house I found a four-foot-tall plastic bunny rabbit with a sign saying 'Happy Easter.' "

"Then," Amy explained to Carol, "Wendy gave me an Easter basket full of real baby chickens. He spent most of his Easter vacation building a chicken coop for them."

"Say, Amy," Kent asked, "whatever did happen to all those chickens?"

"Well . . ." Amy paused, gazing suspiciously at the drumstick in Kent's hand. "Don't worry, Kent. We gave them to an uncle of mine who has a farm in East Texas."

Nibbling daintily at a potato chip, Carol asked Kent between bites, "Are you going to get a job for the summer?"

"Yeah. I hope to work as a counselor at Sky Ranch." He stopped to swallow a bite and dab at his mouth with a paper napkin. "Wendy's going to apply too. It's a terrific camp. Have you ever been there?"

"No, but I've heard it's really a neat place. Won't you have to teach the kids a lot of religious stuff, or something?"

"Yeah," he admitted with a mischievous grin, "but that's a cinch with Wendy around!"

Wendy paused between bites and blushed a deep red.

"I'm sorry, Wen," Kent laughed. "I was only kidding."

"Oh, that's okay, Kent. Maybe it's a good thing *one* of us knows something about religion anyway!"

"Ooooh! Touche'!" Kent groaned. "Seriously, Carol, Sky is a Christian camp and they do study the Bible, but Wendy is pretty sharp on all that . . . I didn't mean to embarrass you, Wendy."

Wendy wiped the chicken crumbs from his fingers and reached for a cupcake. "Don't worry about it. I'm not really embarrassed. Being a Christian is the most natural thing in the world to me. I just wouldn't want anyone else to think I'm weird or anything."

"Oh, I don't think that at all," Carol assured him. "In fact, I'm very much interested. My family is Catholic, even though we haven't gone to mass very much since I was a little girl . . . but I've always wondered about other faiths. Like . . . in our churches, we have pictures and a crucifix showing Jesus on the cross. But in Protestant churches, there are only plain crosses. You never see Christ on the cross at all. How come?"

Wendy thought for a minute, "I think it's because the whole emphasis of our faith is on an empty cross and Jesus Christ as a risen, living Saviour."

"Hmmm."

Amy was curious too. "What is the significance of the crucifix in your church?"

"Well," Carol answered thoughtfully, "I think maybe they emphasize Christ's sacrifice more. Actually, though, we both accept His death and resurrection."

"That's true," Amy agreed. But I always thought Catholics believed more in Mary than in Christ."

"Oh, no. The Virgin Mary is one of many saints."

"Why are so many prayers directed to her?" Amy asked.

"We believe she has direct access to Christ, even above all the other saints because she is His mother."

Wendy interrupted, "I think that's the main difference, Carol. Protestants believe we can have direct communication with Jesus. In fact, that's the most exciting part to me—to be a part of Him—it really means *being alive in Christ,* allowing His Spirit to live now, through me!"

"We believe we receive the Holy Spirit too, when we are confirmed, but I'm not sure I understand what you mean by 'alive in Christ,'" Carol admitted.

"Well," Wendy tried to explain, "it's like His love flowing through us—like energy! I believe that when we allow Christ into our hearts to be our personal Saviour, the Holy Spirit comes to live within us. Then we are baptized as a symbol of our own death and resurrection. That means we'll never really die. Our bodies will, but our souls—our 'real lives'—are secure right now because He lives and loves us."

Carol grinned knowingly at Kent. "I'm beginning to see what you mean, Kent."

"Right!" he agreed, patting Wendy on the shoulder. "We won't have any trouble at Sky Ranch."

They laughed together easily. Wendy blushed again, but Amy came to his rescue quickly. "I admire you, Wendy, for knowing just what you believe. Some of us go to church all our lives without ever stopping to consider what we actually believe and what Christ means to us personally."

Kent spoke up, "I can tell you what I believe . . . I believe we're all much too serious!"

Carol proceeded to stuff an egg in Kent's mouth. Then he and Wendy had a race to finish off the rest of the cupcakes.

"I don't think I can get up!" Wendy groaned at last.

"Me, either," Kent agreed. "In fact, you may have to carry me home in the *back* of the truck. I'll never be able to squeeze into the cab after all that food."

It was after three o'clock when the girls realized they should be getting home and Kent regretfully remembered he was supposed to mow the lawn.

While Carol gathered up the last remains of their feast, Kent leaned back against a tree and watched Wendy and Amy as they walked hand in hand down the hill. He thought to himself how perfect they were together, each so sensitive to the other's feelings and emotions. Amy was always ready with a word or a glance to bolster Wendy's ego, to reinforce his confidence. Kent wondered silently why he suddenly felt so strangely uneasy about them.

Carol shook out the blanket and folded it, then came over to sit beside him. Following his gaze, she said, "They're getting pretty serious, aren't they?"

"Ummm," he answered thoughtfully. "I think they could be, but then Wendy's pretty serious about everything he does . . . I just hope . . ."

"You just hope what?"

"Oh, I just hope we'll always be friends. He has so much going for him, so much future ahead of him, and he moves so fast . . . I don't know what I'd do without him to keep me on the right track."

"Of course you'll always be friends! I think you're just a little bit jealous," Carol teased. "Don't worry about Amy. Why, nothing in the whole world could ever come between you and Wendy!"

2.

Hyacinth blossoms! Beautiful, lavender-colored hyacinths lined the walk in front of the house. Kent remembered watching Wendy and his Mom plant the bulbs over two years ago. But they hadn't bloomed in the spring. Wendy had grinned and explained simply, "God isn't ready yet! He decides when He wants His flowers to bloom!"

On the night of the drill-team party, Wendy was so full of butterflies he could almost have walked on the ceiling. Kent took one look at him and said, "It's a good thing I'm driving. You look like you swallowed a moth!"

Although he would never have admitted it, Kent felt a little queasy himself. To Wendy, though, Kent was always the epitome of cool confidence. He could come up with a wisecrack in any situation to put everyone at ease quickly. Most of all, he seemed to know instinctively what others were feeling. Though he was an incurable tease, he never failed to be a real friend, and Wendy was grateful and admired him for it.

But that night, even Kent's soothing charm didn't help as Wendy knocked at Amy's front door. One look at her in a flowing blue dress, her brown hair curling softly about her face, and his knees turned to rubber. He shoved the plastic box of flowers awkwardly into her hand and tried not to stare. She thanked him shyly and flashed a smile that, all at once, made her nose crinkle, her eyes turn soft and shiny, and his heart jump.

Somehow they made it to the car and Wendy slid into the back seat after her with an audible sigh of relief. His confidence began to return with the roar of the engine and the knowledge that it was Kent's turn at bat.

While Kent went up to Carol's front door, Wendy made a clumsy attempt at conversation. "It's a pretty night, isn't it?" he said, "I mean, warm and all."

"Yes, it really is," Amy agreed. "Wendy, I'm very glad you're taking me tonight. I know you didn't want to, really, but I just didn't want to go with anyone but you."

"Oh, it wasn't that I didn't want to go with you—I really did! It's just that I get . . . so . . ."

"Uptight?"

"Yes, I guess so."

"I know what you mean. But, once we're there, I think you'll enjoy it. We spent all afternoon at the gym," she went on reassuringly, "blowing up balloons and hanging crepe paper streamers. It looks terrific! You'll be surprised."

"It sounds great," Wendy answered, trying to sound confident.

At that moment Kent reappeared and made a dashing gesture of opening the car door for his date.

"Oh, Carol, you look just beautiful!" Amy cried.

Carol squeezed into the front seat, surrounded by tons of billowing green fabric, a delicate corsage of white carnations, and mounds of shining auburn hair swinging loosely down her back. Suddenly they were all chattering at once in anxious anticipation.

The party was a glittering success. The gym was beautifully decorated, as Amy had promised, and the entertainment was enjoyable—not to talk about the endless Cokes and cookies. Before he realized it, Wendy was laughing and actually enjoying himself. "Hey," he whispered in Amy's ear as she sat beside him, "I'm awfully glad I came."

"Me, too," Amy agreed, gazing up at him with soft, brown velvet eyes. For a minute he felt lightheaded under the spell of those luminous eyes, rimmed with dark, curved lashes.

They sat close together, talking almost in each other's ears.

"Are you sure you're glad?" Wendy asked.

"I'm sure," Amy answered solemnly. "Somehow I feel very special when I'm with you."

"Maybe that's because *you are* special!" he whispered.

Wendy's fantasy dissolved and reality returned abruptly as there was a brief pause in the music. The moment slipped past unnoticed by everyone but Amy, who was keenly aware of the flush on Wendy's cheeks and the racing of her own heart. Wisely, she said nothing, but the look in her eyes and the touch of her hand on his spoke clearly.

Kent and Carol reappeared with four soft drinks in paper cups. Carol sat down and caught Kent's arm, pulling him down onto a chair beside her. Yet, five minutes later, Kent was up again attracting a large audience with his comical imitations of the football coaches.

Before they realized it, the evening was gone. It was past midnight when the four of them collapsed into the car. They had to hurry to Kip's for ice cream and still get the girls home before their special one o'clock deadline.

Saturday morning at nine o'clock, right on schedule, Wendy was shaking Kent awake, reminding him that spring had brought them more than "love." Along with the warm weather, came extra chores for both boys. There were tons of leaves to be raked, flower beds to be worked and seeds to be planted. The boys decided the work would go faster if they helped each other.

"We'll start at my house this week and do yours next week," Kent suggested.

"Oh, yeah? And who voted on that arrangement?" Wendy demanded quickly.

Finally a coin toss settled the dispute and they did start at Kent's house after all, working all day Saturday and a couple of evenings during the week after practice. Kent's parents were very pleased with the results and paid the boys for their efforts.

Wendy's yard the following week took longer. There were so many leaves, it took hours just to rake them all. On Saturday they tackled the flower beds which stretched around the house and along either side of the front walk. At noon, Wendy's Mom brought them a pitcher of lemonade and a plate full of sandwiches.

"Hey, things are really taking shape," she exclaimed. "I'm sure the jonquils and daffodils are grateful to have all those leaves cleared from around them."

"Look over there, Mom, your azalea buds are just about to burst open."

"Oh, they're going to be beautiful this year," she said proudly.

"Say," Kent interrupted, swallowing half a cheese sandwich in one gulp, "what happened to all those 'hyabrids,' or whatever they were that you planted?"

A puzzled expression clouded Jo Hickman's face.

Wendy laughed and explained, "Hyacinths! I think he means hyacinths."

"Oh—here they are," Jo laughed, pointing to some thick green sprouts protruding from the soft earth beside the walk. "I can't understand why they aren't blooming. Hyacinths are usually the first ones."

"Mom," Wendy teased, "God isn't ready yet. Don't you know that He decides when He wants His flowers to bloom? And they won't until He tells them to!"

Jo and Kent had to laugh at the simple truth of Wendy's statement, not realizing then the full significance of it. Reluctantly the boys finished the last of the sandwiches and returned to their labor.

There was still more to do when they quit at four o'clock, deciding unanimously that the rest of the flower beds would wait until the next Saturday, but the girls, who were expecting them at six, would not. They might have accomplished even more had they not spent the better part of an hour watching the antics of a red bird in the yard next door.

It was rather unusual activity for a cardinal. He was flitting back and forth between a tall oak tree and a green station wagon parked in the neighbor's drive. The bird stayed around most of the afternoon, leaving only when the curious boys ventured too close. They searched the trees nearby, but couldn't spot a nest, or anything to demand such loyal attention from the beautiful scarlet-plumed bird.

Several times during the week following, Wendy again noticed the cardinal engaged in some mysteriously frantic activity in the neighbor's yard. Jo, too, had become intrigued with the mystery and joined the boys in their observations.

"Cardinals almost always stay together in pairs," she reported to Wendy on Thursday. "But I've never seen the female."

"Maybe he's a confirmed bachelor!" Wendy offered.

"Oh, you!"

"Do you think he's building a nest somewhere nearby?"

"That would be the most natural thing, of course, but I've never seen him pick up any string, or grass. Most birds this time of year are obviously gathering materials for a nest. This one seems to be so agitated about something, he's forgotten what he's supposed to be doing."

"Every time I see him, he's hopping around on that car," Wendy said. "Something about it certainly seems to fascinate him."

Saturday morning, Wendy and Kent decided to settle the mystery once and for all. They took a couple of crates from the storage room and set up a makeshift blind behind the cedar shrubs at the front corner of the house. As inconspicuously as possible, they wedged into their narrow enclosure, peering over the bushes, to watch and wait.

They didn't have to wait long before the cardinal appeared and, without so much as a glance in their direction, began his agitated dance on the hood of the station wagon.

"Look at that!" Kent whispered. "He looks like he's showing off for an audience."

The boys stared in amazement as the brightly plumed bird strutted about, tilting his head majestically and ruffling his neck feathers until it looked as if he might burst with pride.

Wendy spoke softly, "Do you suppose he's establishing his territory? Maybe he's warning other birds to keep away?"

"Sure . . . He's probably staking a claim on that Ford Country Squire because he's tired of flying and wants to drive for a while!" Kent snickered, punching his friend in the ribs playfully.

Wendy's reflexes reacted sharply and he jerked aside; the packing crate collapsed sideways and dumped him heavily onto the ground. All the noise and laughter startled the redbird who chirped angrily at the interruption and took off in a flurry.

A few minutes later Mrs. Taylor came out of the house next door and drove off in the car. The boys reluctantly went back to work putting the flower beds in order and setting out some bedding plants, under Jo's artistic supervision.

Every so often throughout the afternoon, Wendy stopped to look for their feathered friend, but it was only after the car had returned to the drive several hours later, that he finally spotted the bird again.

"Hey, there he is!"

As eager to solve the mystery as they were to take a break from their chores, Wendy and Kent paused to watch the bird's antics once more.

"There he goes again," Kent whispered. The perky redbird was already busy with his mysterious dance beside the rearview mirror which was mounted on the left front fender of the car's hood. Suddenly Kent grabbed Wendy's arm, "It's the mirror, Wen! Look! He sees himself in the rearview mirror!"

"Why, what a conceited little rascal! He's admiring himself."

Both boys watched in amazement as the cardinal preened and fluttered his feathers, oblivious to everything else around him. He cocked his head first one way, then the other, dancing around and around, but always keeping an eye on his reflection in the glass.

"Do you suppose he thinks it's another bird, and he's challenging him?" Wendy asked thoughtfully.

"Maybe. . . . Or, maybe he's in love?" Kent suggested.

Wendy was very touched by the whole incident with the cardinal. He told Amy about it a few days later. "It seems like such a strange thing for a bird to spend so much time like that, just admiring himself, when he should be building his nest, or something constructive."

"I guess he's never seen himself before," Amy said, "and the sight just fascinated him."

"Mom told me today that Mrs. Taylor is going to take the mirror off her car because her fender's getting so scratched up."

"Oh . . . I feel kind of sorry for him," Amy admitted. "I wonder what he will think, when he can't see himself anymore?"

"Maybe it's just as well. Now, he can get back to his family, or whatever. . . . You know, there are a lot of people who, just like that redbird, spend so much of their lives staring at an image of themselves, that they miss out on what the world is really all about. I guess we're all guilty of that sometimes."

"You mean being selfish and thinking only of ourselves?"

"Yeah, but more than that. Just like that bird 'fell in love' with his own reflection in the mirror and couldn't resist staring at it, maybe we sometimes get so wrapped up in ourselves, we miss out on the opportunities that are in front of us. Am I making any sense?"

"Yes," Amy answered with a solemn expression, "but please don't throw out all the mirrors just yet. I'm not sure I'm ready to give them up 'cold cardinal'!"

"Oh, brother," Wendy groaned.

Tuesday night there was to be a regional meeting of the Fellowship of Christian Athletes. By Monday, Wendy was in a terrible state. He had agreed to speak on the program; he'd even decided to tell the story of the cardinal and explain how the FCA organization encourages young men and women to allow their lives to reflect the Spirit of Christ in the world, and not just their own desires. He read his whole speech out loud to Kent, ending with a comparison between a football team that depends on every player's talents and strong coaching, and a team where each player wants to carry the ball and ignores the coach's instructions.

When Wendy finished reading, he crumpled the paper and tossed it against the wall with a grunt of disgust.

"Hey, what's the big idea? It's a terrific speech!" Kent shouted.

"Oh, it's dumb! I don't know why I ever got myself into this. Who wants to hear about a stupid old nearsighted bird?"

"Wendy, for pete's sake, calm down. You're not exactly campaigning for the Senate, you know. It's just a little speech. I thought it sounded pretty good."

"Thanks, Kent, but you're my best friend. Anyway, even if the dumb speech is okay, I'll never be able to do it. I'm already shaking, just thinking about it!"

"Hey, Bozo, aren't you the one that's always telling me to depend on God? All those heroes you talk about in the Bible were probably more scared than you are, but God helped them, didn't He? And since you're always making such a point of it to the rest of us, I don't think He's likely to let His number one press agent down, do you?"

Wendy mustered a weak smile. "Thanks, Kent. You're right. I know the Lord will hold me up once I'm in front of all those people. And maybe, He'll even make my mouth work. It's getting my legs to take me up there I'm most worried about."

Tuesday night, Wendy was still scared stiff. Kent was torn between concern for his friend and amusement that it was Wendy for a change who was suffering from self-doubt. When it was time, Wendy stepped up and started slowly and shakily, but the more he talked, the calmer he became. It wasn't exactly the same speech he had read to Kent; it was actually better. By the time he had finished, Wendy was smiling confidently. Kent was truly amazed.

Later, on the way home, they talked about it.

"Wendy, you were so cool. I can't believe it! It wasn't even the same speech."

"I can't believe it either!" Wendy admitted. "Once I got started I forgot about myself, and I guess God really did take over."

"Aw, come on, Wendy! This is Kent you're talkin' to."

"It's really like the cardinal, Kent. I found out you can't just look at yourself. When you ask for help, you have to look up and see the rest of the world. When I got up to talk I was so scared I *had* to let go. I just put it in God's hands and prayed, 'Lord, I can't do this. Please help me!' It was only when I really stopped worrying about what people would think of *me,* and how *I* was going to look to them, that I started to relax and think clearly. My thoughts seemed to come easier and God could help me know what I should say. And, the more at ease I felt, the better I felt about sharing my feelings."

"That sounds simple enough, but it's really kind of heavy on the spiritual stuff, Wendy. I'm just not that spiritual, I guess. But I'm not a very good Christian either. When I have a chance to speak up, I get all tongue-tied. I'm afraid I usually let God down. I can't seem to do anything right except on the football field!"

"Let me ask you something, Kent. Do you believe that God made us and gave us the talents we have, even for football?"

"Yeah, I guess so."

"Well, do you think He goofed? Or, is it possible He made us, just as we are, with talents *and* faults, for His own purposes? So that His power can work *through our* weaknesses?"

"Yeah, maybe. But wouldn't it be easier if He had just made us perfect to begin with?"

"That's the whole point, Kent. He made us all individuals with freedom of choice. We can use our talents and our weaknesses any way we choose. We can waste them like the cardinal was doing, or we can choose to have Christ live through us. Actually the less we have to start with, the more His strength can work through us.

"You were right last night when you reminded me of the 'Heroes' in the Bible," Wendy continued. "I read again about Moses late last night. When God spoke to him and told him to lead the Israelites out of

Egypt, he gave the Lord all kinds of excuses why he couldn't do the job. First, he said he wasn't the right person to go. He figured they would hate him because he had grown up in Pharaoh's palace. Second, he didn't know what to say to the people. And, they wouldn't believe him anyway. Next, he argued that he was such a poor speaker; he was even handicapped by a speech impediment! And last, in desperation, he begged to be excused because he was afraid."

"Wow!" Kent retorted. "I sure didn't know all that!"

"Yes, and Moses thought he just couldn't do what God asked," Wendy went on, "and yet, Moses became a great leader because God worked through him, using even those weaknesses to accomplish His own purposes."

"I'm convinced," Kent answered in amazement. "I guess if Moses was afraid and doubted, then maybe it's not so surprising that we feel the same way. I think I'd like to read that myself."

"Good! Why don't you? It's in the second and third chapters of Exodus. Wait'll you read the part about the snake—it'll blow your mind."

"Snake—what snake?"

"Oh, no! You'll have to look it up for yourself to find out what God asked Moses to do next!"

3

Every time he looked up and saw a very bright star twinkling in the sky, Kent would remember Wendy's words, "I think people are a lot like stars, Kent. God places us just where He wants us and then it's up to us to shine as brightly as we can. All we really are is reflectors. The more we absorb God's Spirit, the brighter we begin to glow."

There was an easy sort of friendly atmosphere in Wendy's home. That's probably why Kent spent so much time there. He felt he could talk to Wendy's Mom and Dad about anything in the world. Wendy realized it too, and told him why he thought his family was so special. It was how they felt about each other and their lives together. Kent could sense the warmth when he was there. They weren't "religious" in the sense you normally use the word. It was a very natural attitude. They had a very personal feeling about God and they talked so easily about Christ you got the feeling He was a real and close friend.

Wendy's dad was an enigma to Kent. Solidly built, with thinning, sandy-colored hair, he remained perennially young by virtue of a boyishly innocent grin, and a mischievous twinkle in his eye. A self-made man, both successful and unpretentious, he approached life as a game to be won and enjoyed, but never taken too seriously.

There were no limits to the horizons he encouraged his sons to explore. Wendy told Kent how, when he was fourteen and Andy only thirteen, his Dad took them twenty miles across the sprawling Dallas Metroplex, gave them each a five dollar bill, and told them to find their own way home, by any means at their disposal! Bob Hickman believed in preparing his sons to face the world with confidence and eagerness.

Although he provided more than adequately for his family's needs, the boys were expected to contribute as well. In addition to their chores at home, they often cut lawns, washed cars, and during the summer, delivered fruit baskets for the Goodman Produce Company.

Kent soon learned that being around the Hickmans meant being success-oriented. While Bob encouraged a strict training program which included high protein diets, calisthenics and supervised weight lifting, Wendy's Mom provided her own training ground in impeccable good manners and a genuine concern for the feelings of others.

Jo Hickman was an artist and a very talented lady. Petite and graceful, she looked much more like an artist's model than the master of the brush. Kent admired her beautiful paintings, and the warm, comfortable atmosphere she had created in their home. But most of all, he admired her ability to see through all the outward pretenses and recognize inside of people the traits that really matter. She was straightforward, even blunt, often forcing Kent to look at himself more honestly than he had ever dared.

Lavish with her affection and her criticism, when she felt it was called for, she casually ignored the trivial and chose to be concerned only with what she determined to be the essential qualities of life.

Once Kent remarked that Jo Hickman was ten percent human, ten percent angel, and eighty percent sense of humor. Still, you could never be certain which part was in control at a given moment. She was unpredictable in many ways, yet invariably honest. He knew instinctively that she was a friend he could count on for the truth. Perhaps even more than anyone in his own family, he valued her opinion and advice.

Andy was bright and enthusiastic, following Wendy like a shadow. With his Father's zest for life and a strong measure of his Mother's sensitivity, he was somehow less intense than his brother. In a difficult situation, Wendy was inclined to retreat within himself until he'd worked out a solution, while Andy found it easier to seek and accept the guidance of others.

Each of the boys shared with Bob a natural serenity, sharply evident in Andy's gentle nature and only softly muted by Wendy's rugged determination.

While each of the Hickmans contributed his own unique quality to the family, it was far from being a perfect balance. When four strong individuals share the same roof, there are bound to be conflicts. But seeing how they worked out the difficulties and depended on God to hold them together, was a lesson in love Kent would always remember.

Christ really was the center of Wendy's family. This notion might have seemed unusual under other circumstances, but it was so natural and easy in their home that it never dawned on Kent to question it. He merely respected and even envied them.

On many weekends the Hickmans invited a whole group of kids for a camping trip. They would start early packing sleeping bags, water skis and a basket filled with hot dogs, mustard, buns and chili in the back of their pickup truck.

Just as they thought everything was ready, someone would yell, "Did anybody pack the stuff to make 'smores'?"

Suddenly eight or ten heads would pop out of the truck to look hopefully at Wendy's Mom who invariably smiled and held up a paper sack in answer to their questioning looks.

"Smores" were definitely the best invention yet for camping! First, they needed a cool night, a blazing campfire, lots of songs and laughter and any gang of kids. Then all it took was toasted marshmallows placed between pieces of chocolate bars and graham crackers, and everyone was suddenly saying, "How 'bout s'more?"

After just such a happy evening, when everyone had crawled into his sleeping bag full and content, the camp at last grew quiet and hushed under a glistening canopy of stars.

"Hey, Wendy," Kent said loudly, his voice echoing in the darkness, "I'm sure glad Andy is finally grown up enough to sleep by himself now. Aren't you?"

They both laughed at Andy's muffled groans remembering a Boy Scout camp several years before when Andy had felt suddenly homesick and frightened, and Wendy got up in the middle of the night and carried his sleeping bag into the tent to be close to him. Kent remembered the sound of his quiet voice in the stillness telling Andy not to be afraid, that he was right there and that God was always looking out for him. Andy gradually stopped sobbing and reached for his brother's hand in the darkness. "I love you, Wendy," he whispered.

"I love you, too," Wendy answered.

Now as they lay stretched out beside the last warm embers of the campfire, Kent listened to Wendy talking softly while the stars twinkled above them.

"I think people are a lot like stars, Kent. God places us just where He wants us and then it's up to us to shine as brightly as we can. We are really only reflectors. The more we absorb God's Spirit, the brighter we begin to glow."

"I'm not sure how much of God's Spirit I have," Kent admitted. "I still let myself get in the way too often and depend on what I can do instead of letting the Lord take over. How do you manage to keep Him in charge of things?"

"Oh, I forget too. But I keep reminding myself that all the good things in my life are there because He put them there. And when something is wrong, it's usually because I moved without Him."

"But how can you be sure what God wants you to do?"

Wendy was quiet for a minute. "When I have a problem or a decision to make, I've found God helps me through His Word. I try to pray and read the Bible every day. It may sound corny, but it isn't. We work so hard practicing and getting ready for football. Well, talking to God and studying His Book are just exercises to strengthen our faith. Besides, I honestly enjoy it.

"As I've said before, I think of the Bible as a great adventure filled with heroes who are people just like you and me, but who were constantly striving to win the world for God. But it's the end that counts. No adventure would be complete without a happy ending, and the ending of the Bible, and of our lives on this earth, is Jesus Christ. We, as Christians, should recognize that He is the answer to our problems and the beginning of our real, true happiness. Right?"

"I know that's true, Wendy. I only wish I had as much faith as you."

"Hey, Kent, it's easy to lie here in the dark and talk about faith. But you and I both know how hard it is when the problems come from all directions in the middle of the day. That's why I'm grateful for a friend like you to share things with."

During a couple of rainy days, uncharacteristic for June, the boys tore down the motors on their go-carts and rebuilt them entirely. The very next week, Kent was down with a sore throat. A little penicillin soon had him back on his feet, and by Friday he was climbing the walls to get outside again. So he jumped at the chance when Wendy telephoned, "Wanna take the go-carts down to the park and try them out?"

"You bet! I'll be right over."

They walked to the park, pulling the carts behind them. Smiling and talking a mile a minute, Wendy sounded especially happy and full of bright expectations.

"You know what I'd like to have someday, Kent? A jeep. A fire-engine red four-wheel drive. We could just take off and go anywhere! A jeep'll run through water, over ditches, and just about any place you'd want to go. Someday, Kent, that's what we'll do!"

Kent laughed at his sudden determination, never doubting for a moment that his friend would succeed wherever that determination led him.

All morning they raced the go-carts in and around the bumpy park trails, the raspy roar of engines drowning out the rest of the world. Sitting only a foot off the ground on wooden planks with four wheels attached, they bounced up and down like popcorn with every dip, legs braced against the footboard and hands gripping the wheel more tightly with each twisting curve.

At last, when the gas supply was depleted, they walked back, pulling the carts along behind them. Wendy interrupted the brief solitude by asking, "Are you all packed and ready to go?"

"Yeah, pretty much. Mom's still fussing that I won't have enough socks. If she had her way, I'd probably need a U-haul trailer to get all my junk to camp. Is your Dad still planning to take us out there?"

"Yes. He's planning to leave Sunday afternoon about three. That will give us time to see Mike Albin and find out what our schedule is like."

The boys had applied as summer camp counselors at Sky Ranch. On the application form they were asked to write a brief biographical sketch. Wendy wrote easily of his home, of camping trips with his

Dad and his brother, Andy. Kent was very touched by Wendy's special tribute to his Mom, and his simple testimony of faith:

> *"I can say with complete honesty that my homelife is spiritually stimulated with the Word of God. I believe it is my mother who has contributed far above her responsibilities to raise two boys in a family of four. Only second to Christ Himself, I feel I can turn to my mother for complete reassurance in the things I do.*
>
> *"Without this reassurance in both Christ and life itself, any family, no matter how complete it may seem, will gradually separate at the seams. Any family member who hopes to lead a wholesome life must be assured that Christ can be a stepping-stone out of our problems if we put our trust in Him."*

Sky Ranch turned out to be a fantastic experience for both boys. In a beautiful wooded area just out of Denton, Texas, it offered everything for young campers: swimming, sailing, canoeing, horsemanship, archery, riflery and crafts, all sponsored by a nondenominational Christian faculty.

As counselors, Kent and Wendy were in charge of a cabin of ten boys. It was kind of a switch to have kids asking them so many questions. They both grew very close to the younger guys, helping them learn about horses or sailing during the day and having long talks at bedtime about their problems or anxieties. As their charges learned, Wendy and Kent found themselves growing closer to the Lord, too.

They read the Bible each morning and prayed together. In the evening they talked about what they were learning and tried to answer questions. After the boys were tucked away in bed, the counselors would get together in the trading post for Cokes and discuss any problems that had come up.

One night, Kent was anxious to get to the trading post early because of a blonde counselor from one of the girls' cabins he had met. His plan worked perfectly. First he read to the boys from Genesis the story of Adam and Eve, ending with God's command in the 28th verse, "Be fruitful, multiply, and replenish the earth."

"Now, if you guys have any questions, Wendy here will be glad to answer them. I have some important business at the camp office. See you later!"

Without another word, he dashed out the door, leaving a shocked Wendy, mouth gaping, as ten small boys waited eagerly for an explanation of God's plan for replenishing the earth!

After a vacation trip with her parents, Amy joined the boys at Sky Ranch as a counselor for the twelve-year-old girls. She rode out with Kent one afternoon, after he had been home for a weekend off, bombarding him with questions all the way. "How does Wendy really like it? Is he great with the kids? Do you think he'll be glad to see me? Do the counselors have many chances to get together? Did you tell him what time we'd be there? How much farther is it?"

Kent just shook his head and tried to squeeze in an answer now and then. She stopped suddenly as they pulled into the camp parking area at last and caught sight of Wendy coming toward them.

Before Kent could even stop the car, Amy jumped out and ran to meet him. As he maneuvered into a parking space, he glanced in the rearview mirror in time to see Wendy wrap his arms around her. Kent smiled and thought to himself, "Well, I don't think he'll be needing my advice any longer. He seems to have matters well in hand."

Sky meant many new experiences for Kent and Wendy. They made new friendships and learned a great deal about themselves as well.

That's where they met Tom. He was a unit director in charge of their cabin and three others. Although he was a little older, they quickly discovered how much they had in common. While Tom shared Wendy's strong sense of responsibility and integrity, it was soon obvious that he also had Kent's flair for getting entangled in mischief.

Of course, pranks were common among the counselors, but the aftereffects were usually of briefer duration than one particular evening's adventure.

It began innocently enough as the three boys sat perched on the Ping-Pong table at the edge of the grassy recreation field. Tom first noticed the two girls walking casually along the path toward the bathhouse. "They must have just come from my cabin," he said, as a vague suspicion began to dawn upon him. "It's the only one in that direction. They've done something! I'll go see what shape my cabin's in—you two, stop them and hold them till I get back!"

"Okay, but be careful. You can't tell what they've been up to."

Wendy and Kent took off, going in the opposite direction from Tom, and circled around the bathhouse to apprehend the suspects.

The startled girls were the picture of wide-eyed innocence. The boys stood firm and accusing, the girls denying with nervous giggles and furtive glances.

When Tom reached the cabin, he peered cautiously through the window. It looked quiet and deserted. Carefully, he pushed open the door, half expecting a bucket of water to come splashing down. When nothing happened, he ventured further inside.

The cabin was empty and in its normally cluttered order. There were no tacks on the floor, or rocks in the suitcase. There was no soap in his sneakers, no syrup on the doorknobs, or garbage under the bed. "The bed! They just might . . . !"

Tom threw back the cover and frowned at his sheets covered with a two-inch layer of sand!

A plan of revenge immediately began to form in his thoughts. Quickly he grabbed a metal container from a zippered bag in the corner and dashed out the door. He hurried back up the path toward the showers, ready to convict and punish the offenders. But the girls heard him coming, and elected to run. Wendy and Kent in startled pursuit caught one of them, but discovered her so difficult to hold that the other one escaped.

Tom arrived breathless but relishing his moment of revenge. Oblivious to her screams and struggles, they covered her with shaving cream from head to toe. In fact, they became so absorbed in their project they failed to notice the rescue squad approaching in the darkness, their aerosol weapons loaded and ready.

Ten minutes later the battle scene resembled a clip from a horror film, with seven of the stickiest, dirtiest "creatures" anyone could have invented.

When all the shaving cream had been sufficiently smeared, someone in desperation resorted to a handful of sand. Thus began the gritty storm which led to the predicament of the grimy creatures at the timely arrival of the adult sponsors.

The laughter and screams had turned to choking and gasping, and the fun was definitely over!

However, the saddest part was yet to come with the announcement that a plumbing problem had developed a few hours earlier and the showers were "out of order"!

Since there was a positive rule against swimming after dark, it seemed only a fitting punishment that the "sticky creatures" must endure until the morrow.

The fame of that escapade followed the boys for quite some time.

The three were inseparable that summer. But it wasn't all fun and pranks. Their first priority was helping their young charges. Of course, there were occasions when they temporarily misplaced those priorities.

At one point, Mike, as ranch director, decided that his counselors were growing lax about their evening duties. At ten p.m. all campers were required to be in their cabins ready for evening devotionals. Yet, there were always at least a dozen counselors in the trading post at the very time they were supposed to be holding cabin programs.

As it happened, Wendy and Amy were both there at the moment Mike elected to "chew them out." Properly reprimanded the transgressors lost little time getting back to their appointed duties. However, later in the evening, one of them came alone to the office where Mike and Tom were still working, to apologize and assure them that the responsibility would never again be taken lightly. It was Wendy, with tears in his eyes. He told them how much he cared about the younger boys and how he wanted them to have a chance to know Jesus Christ as he did. They prayed together and asked God's help in directing their own lives and those who looked to them for guidance.

After camp was over Wendy continued to write to Tom, sharing some of the discoveries he made from his own study of the Bible. He wrote sincerely of his faith in words unusually mature for a sixteen-year-old.

> *"I have discovered a truly great verse in Isaiah 60:19. It speaks of how we are to let our everlasting light shine. Another verse,*

Isaiah 59:16, says: 'He saw no one was helping you, and wondered that no one intervened. Therefore, He Himself, stepped in to save you through His mighty power and justice.'

"The Lord is really some kind of guy to do all that for you and me!"

"Isaiah 57:1,2 talks about why such good and kind people die, sometimes even at an early age. The answer is most logical. 'The good men perish; the godly die before their time and no one seems to care or wonder why. No one seems to realize that God is taking them away from evil days ahead. For the godly who die shall rest in peace.'

"I must close now and please forgive me for not writing sooner. I will be praying for you, Tom.

May God bless you
Your friend and brother in Christ,
Wendy

P. S. Smile, God loves you—and me too!"

It was a beautiful summer for Kent and Wendy. They had grown physically and spiritually. Kent had matured too. He had taken part in the devotions at camp, read the Bible and explained to the boys how to trust Christ as their Saviour, but still he felt himself holding back. Somehow, he couldn't quite trust God with everything. After all, he convinced himself, "God helps those who help themselves."

Even as he thought it, he could hear the echo of Wendy's words, "Someday, Kent, you'll find you can't do it all alone."

4.

It was a special, unforgettable moment to Kent, like a photograph printed indelibly in his mind. As he looked around at the laughing faces, he wished the feeling could last forever. Wendy too, sensed the magic. Try as he might to hold on, it would surely burst like a bubble in the air . . . .

Most of the boys' time was occupied with school and football workouts. Long, hard sessions of exercise and practice left little energy or incentive for other activities. Skyline was a new high school, anxious and determined to make its mark in the athletic world.

The boys were ready and eager while the girls were a little less than enthusiastic. The long, strenuous practices, plus the renewal of books and study all meant seeing much less of each other.

Amy, in particular, felt that Wendy's commitment to football often created a sensitive area between them. She resented what she considered his "typically male" attitude, expecting total loyalty from her while anything related to sports automatically took precedence over their private plans. She usually managed to hide her feelings, afraid that any negative response might threaten her position in Wendy's life.

He was the most important thing in her world right now. All she really wanted was to know that he felt the same way about her, but in her heart she knew that *everything*, including football, took second place to his faith. And though she tried to understand, this too was hard to accept.

She was delighted when Wendy's Dad suggested a campout over the Labor Day weekend. Until . . .

Saturday dawned hot and still—one of those "Dog Days" as they call them in Texas—at the end of summer when the air is thick and a haze seems to smother the earth under a heavy veil.

That morning a whole caravan of cars gathered at Wendy's house to head for the lake. Sitting in the cab of the pickup, while Wendy packed the last of the gear, Amy felt anything but delighted. Her dream of a quiet weekend together away from everything had blossomed into a giant excursion which included half the football team and their girlfriends.

That's the way it often was with Wendy's family. They believed in that old adage, "the more the merrier"! Any other time, Amy might have agreed, but *not this weekend.* She felt irritable and grumpy, and even more depressed because she knew she was acting like a spoiled, petulant child. She was sorry about it but she couldn't help it. And Wendy's attitude didn't do anything to improve matters; he was being so sweet and understanding, she felt like screaming!

He climbed into the cab beside her and spoke cautiously, "Amy, I'm sorry it didn't work out quite like you wanted, but we'll have a great time. Wait and see. We'll go for a long walk, away from everyone, just you and me . . ."

"Don't try to pacify me, Wendy. I'm not a child. I just didn't realize this was going to be a football retreat!"

Andy and his friend, David, showed up just then to squeeze in with Wendy and Amy. Everyone was packed and ready to go.

"Don't worry, Am," Wendy assured her, squeezing her hand, "there'll be no football *this* weekend."

Only, of course, there was. They had barely unpacked the gear and set up camp before some of the guys were involved in a fast game of "two-below," which is touch-football with the added stipulation that a tackler must touch a runner below the waist with both hands in order to stop the play.

Saturday afternoon was feverish with activities; swimming, water skiing and clowning. By evening everyone was starved and devoured mounds of sandwiches and cookies. They sang every song they could remember, and a few they didn't, and finally collapsed into their sleeping bags with full stomachs and sore muscles.

Sunday morning they held their own brief service around the campfire. Andy read some verses from I Corinthians where Paul compared the Christian's life to that of an athlete and spoke about what he had read:

> *"In a race, everyone runs but only one person gets first prize. So run your race to win. To win the contest you must deny yourselves many things that would keep you from doing your best. An athlete goes to all this trouble just to win a blue ribbon or a silver cup, but we do it for a heavenly reward that never disappears. So I run straight to the goal with purpose in every step. I fight to win. I'm not just shadow-boxing or playing around. Like an athlete I punish my body, treating it roughly, training it to do what it should, not what it wants to. Otherwise, I fear that after enlisting others for the race, I myself might be declared unfit and ordered to stand aside."*

It was easy for all of the kids to identify with the analogy. Most of them were already Christians and understood when Kent attempted to explain his feelings, "I try to live as a Christian should. When I mess things up, I just get up and try again. I think that's all God expects of us. What about you, Jake?"

Jake, a six-foot-two-inch black guard on the team, had sat listening quietly as the others talked. He claimed to be an atheist, just like his father. Once he had told Kent, "Me and my Dad, we don't buy this religious stuff! The only one you can ever count on is you, man, and that's it!" He was usually very quiet and rarely spoke up in a group, but now, challenged by Kent's question, he shook his head. "Sorry, man, but I don't buy it."

Karen offered a feminine point of view, "Although I'm not an athlete, I think being a Christian requires the same kind of dedication. You wouldn't win many games if you ignored all the rules, and being a Christian means a lot more. I think the most important thing to consider is *why* you do either one. If you really love sports, you'll play better.

"Jesus told us that loving God and loving others are the two most important 'rules' for a Christian. It's funny, but, to me, when I think about loving God and caring about others, the 'rules' don't seem so important. It's just a natural way to live."

Wendy agreed with Karen, but he also knew that being an athlete is often very hard. "I love football and I wouldn't trade the time I've spent in athletics for anything! But, sometimes when you've worked and sweated and put everything you've got into it, and you still lose, you begin to wonder why you're doing it! As a Christian, I get frustrated sometimes too because I don't understand why things happen the way they do. Or, maybe I want to do something to help a friend who has a problem and I just bungle it all up. Then, I remember that we're not alone. Jesus promised to be with us always and to help us live in this world. So, even when we think we've lost, we should remember that, as Christians, we've already won the most important race of all—and the prize is eternal life through Christ."

Kent asked Mr. Hickman to close their service with a prayer.

"Dear Heavenly Father," he prayed, "thank you for these young people and for what their spirit and their love can accomplish in this world. Strengthen our faith, Dear Lord, and lift us up when we fail, to try again. Help us to lean upon Jesus Christ as the only stepping-stone from this world into your Kingdom, and allow His love to shine through us each day. In Jesus' name we pray. Amen."

Ten minutes later they were all heading for the water. Wendy and Kent had a bet going. Even fishing had become a competitive sport between the two of them. "If you catch a five-pound bass, I'll wash your car once a week for a month," Wendy promised.

"Better get your chamois ready," Kent said. "I like a lot of polish on the chrome."

Kent and Wade, Wendy and Jake started out in the Hickmans' boat. By noon they had managed to catch only a few small perch and a turtle. Growing exasperated, Kent cast his line closer to the shore and realized too late it was hopelessly entangled on a submerged tree stump.

Not one for patience, he stood up and began to yank, twist, and pop the line in a futile effort to free it. Jake calmly put down his own reel and moved his giant, black hulk over to assist Kent. "Wait a minute," he cautioned. "You gotta use a little finesse!"

Jake leaned expertly out over the boat and began to apply gentle pressure to the six-pound test line, stretching it first one way and then the other. Kent waited only a moment before deciding that Jake's "finesse" wasn't going to work. Unfortunately, he decided to give the line another hard yank just at the moment Jake managed to free it. What happened next was right out of Laurel and Hardy.

Stanley—er, Kent, flew backwards against the side of the boat, landing sprawled on the deck at Wendy's feet. The boat rocked suddenly backward from the force of his weight and pitched Ollie—er, Jake, off balance and over the side, head first! The accompanying splash brought all three in the boat to their feet, very nearly capsizing the entire craft. Wendy reached out quickly to help his friend but miscalculated the weight of a two-hundred-pound guard when wet, and he too tumbled over the side. Kent and Wade took a few minutes to recover from spasms of laughter before they found the ski ladder and put it over the side.

When at last the two were back aboard, Kent apologized profusely to the dripping black giant beside him, "Jake, I'm really so sorry!"

"Kent," Wendy interrupted. "I guess you win!"

"Huh?"

"The bet . . ." Wendy went on. "That's positively the biggest 'black bass' ever pulled out of this lake!"

Wendy and Wade both dissolved in laughter, as a smiling Jake lifted Kent from his feet, still begging apologies, and casually dropped him over the side.

Late that afternoon, one by one, kids began to collapse in heaps around the camp. They were exhausted, sunburned, mosquito-bitten and ravenous. The boys started a fire while the girls made an attempt at getting the meal started. That's where Wendy's Dad took charge. He was a fantastic organizer.

Bob took the utter chaos of twenty-eight kids and assorted groceries and turned it into what appeared to be a simple picnic. A crisis in his hands became a minor problem swiftly solved. As a master at delegating jobs, he quickly placed a hot dog and a clothes hanger in every empty hand. When a shortage of buns was discovered, he tossed Kent his keys and asked him to dash to the small store up the road for more.

"Hey, Jo," Bob called, "do we need anything else?"

"You might pick up another jar of mustard."

"Okay," he answered, handing Kent a ten-dollar bill.

"I'll go along and help," Amy volunteered. She glanced toward Wendy who was so busy unloading ice chests packed with soft drinks he wouldn't miss her for a while.

As Kent started the car, Amy slid in beside him. "I wanted a chance to talk to you, Kent, about Wendy."

"What's wrong?"

"Things just aren't going too well between us," Amy sadly admitted.

"Really? I didn't know. He hasn't said anything to me."

"It's hard to put in words," she went on, close to tears as she gazed out across the lake as they sped by. "It's just that he doesn't seem to have time for me anymore. I feel like he's pulling away from me and I don't know why . . . I've even wondered if his parents might have asked him not to see me. You know their approval is terribly important to him. I can't think of anything else that might explain it. He hasn't said anything at all to you?"

"No . . . but I know his folks think the world of you. Still, I know they don't want Wendy to be serious about *any* girl yet. They might have discussed that with him. Are you sure you aren't just imagining things? You know, with football and school right now, he really has a lot on his mind."

"You could be right, Kent, but somehow, I think it's more than that," Amy insisted.

"Why don't you talk to him about it? Just ask him straight out what's wrong," he suggested.

"I've been trying to but we haven't had five minutes alone in the last week!"

Kent slowed the car to a stop on the gravel area in front of the small store. He turned off the key but didn't get out. Instead, he turned to face her, reaching over to gently squeeze her shoulder. "Amy, I know Wendy cares a great deal for you. He's a very dedicated person. It's like he's in a hurry to do everything at once. Sometimes he is so intent on what he's involved in, we all get kind of left behind."

"How do you hold on to a shooting star, Kent?" Amy asked him, her voice despairing.

"I'm not sure. But I do know if we can, it will be worth the ride. Talk to him, Amy. Tell him how you feel. And try not to worry!"

"Thanks for listening, Kent, I do feel better. Please don't say anything to him about it, okay?"

"You know I won't. Wendy's my best friend, and the two of you have something very special together. He demands so much of himself, sets such an example, maybe . . . maybe, sometimes he expects too much of the rest of us. He just assumes everyone is as determined as he is. But he needs you! Remember that, Amy, and don't let anything trivial come between you."

While Kent went inside for the mustard and buns, Amy waited in the car, brushing a few errant tears from her face. She knew Kent was right about Wendy, but instead of feeling reassured, she sensed a growing fear deep within her that those very qualities she loved in him might be pulling him farther and farther away from her. She wasn't at all sure she could measure up to his expectations. She prayed that she could!

Wendy came to meet them as they drove up at the camp but didn't ask any questions. Instead he took Amy's arm and whispered, "Tonight, I want you beside me every minute!"

Later when the hot dogs and chili had been sufficiently demolished and everyone was toasting marshmallows for "smores," Debi and Karen started a song. Mike produced a guitar and they sang "Harvest Moon," "Deep in the Heart of Texas," and a few other old standards. Then, when Carol dropped a gooey marshmallow down the front of her yellow T-shirt and blushed with embarrassment, Kent led the guys in "The Yellow Rose of Texas," amid a chorus of girlish giggles.

It was a special, unforgettable moment to Kent, like a photograph printed indelibly in his mind. As he looked around at the laughing faces, he wished the feeling could last forever—the warm sense of togetherness and companionship that had drawn them into a tight circle of friendship. It meant a lot to him, more than he could explain to anyone, and he somehow felt that the strength and happiness of that circle would carry him through many difficult times.

Wendy's face was eager and open, Kent thought, as their eyes met. It was a . . . a hungry look, reaching out for all the love and warmth around him. Instinctively, Kent knew that Wendy too sensed the magic, and he felt genuinely pleased that they could share it.

Even Amy was smiling, though he noticed a shadow in her eyes that reminded him how fleeting a moment could be. And try as he might to hold on, it would surely burst like a bubble in the air. Perhaps its very impermanence gave it more value, a rare thing, like the singing of a bird, to be felt and absorbed, but never captured.

Suddenly the bubble did burst and the magic was disrupted as Karen shrieked in alarm. Wriggling free from the ice which Mike had dropped down her back, she chased him wildly across the sandy lakeshore. A moment later there were barefoot kids scampering in all directions in an informal game of tag.

Taking advantage of the diversion, Wendy caught Amy's hand and led her away from the lake and into the cover of the trees which lined the western shore. As the shadows reached out to enclose them, he drew her against him and kissed her. His arms were strong and secure around her waist, and immediately Amy began to surrender all the fears and doubts which had plagued her. For those few brief seconds, she wanted desperately to believe that nothing else mattered, that she could be all Wendy would ever want or need.

But then, he let her go and stepped back to look, not into her eyes, but up at the stars. Even in the gathering darkness, Amy could see that his heart was not with her, but up there, soaring somewhere high in the heavens far beyond her reach. And the sudden realization was like a searing pain inside her.

"I wonder what it's like up there," Wendy said softly, totally unaware of Amy's thoughts. "If the stars are so beautiful from here, shining through a million miles of darkness, how brilliant do you suppose they are up there? Sometimes I think they could be street lights and that's actually heaven spread out above us with highways stretching across the universe. I bet the scientists at NASA would love to discuss that with me, don't you?"

He laughed at his own imaginings and interpreted the small, raspy sound which escaped from Amy's throat as a chuckle of agreement. "Would you like to walk a while?" he asked.

Slowly Amy regained her control and managed to stammer, "I think we'd better go back before they wonder about us."

"Okay. Hey, you're shivering. I guess it's getting cooler than I realized. C'mon, let's get you back near the fire."

Wendy and Amy were together all the next day, but always in a crowd. There was never a time for serious talk. If Amy was quieter than usual, no one seemed to notice.

Once Kent caught Amy's eye, and the question was loud and clear in the expression on his face. "I'm not giving up," she whispered in answer, "not without a fight!"

5.

Wendy had first noticed the bronze plaque in the chapel at Arlington Cemetery and pointed it out to Kent. The words lingered in his mind, "Living, if it is to be worthy of the name, should mean something more than how many years our hearts beat. The length of our lives, or of living, should be measured in happiness, in what we mean to others."

On the Tuesday after Labor Day, it was back to school and football for Wendy and Kent. The first game of the season was a triumph for the Skyline Raiders as they promptly trampled their opponents 28 to 7.

In the second game they ran into more difficulty. With Kent at quarterback, they moved down the field to within twenty yards of the goal. On a quick pass over the center, Kent threw hard and fast. But, out of nowhere, a green jersey came to snatch the ball away from the receiver. The crowd groaned even as the interceptor was buried beneath a pile of red and blue Raider colors.

Coach Miles sent the defense in, telling Wendy to key in on No. 23, a fast-moving back who looked about ten feet tall. At the snap Wendy lowered his head and charged. It was a handoff to No. 23, but Wendy was right on him. The collision knocked them both sideways and the ball tumbled free just as the whistle blew.

Wendy staggered to his feet, trying to determine why there were so many bells ringing, and if he was late for something. With the help of a teammate he made it safely to the bench where the manager hurried to put ice on his head.

For a minute Wendy felt dazed and confused but he pushed away the ice bag. "I'm okay," he muttered.

Suddenly it all rushed back to him. He jumped to his feet and yelled, "Hey, did we get it back?"

Kent had been standing by, anxious about his friend's injury. Now he laughed out loud and retorted, "No, dummy! You were taking a nap when you should've been grabbing the ball."

Kent never tired of teasing his friend, but underneath he respected and admired him. Once he had overheard Coach Breckenridge tell someone, "Wendy's the hardest worker I've ever seen! Even in practice, he puts everything he's got into it."

Even Coach Miles had once admonished the team in exasperation, "If every one of you guys would work as hard as Wendy, we'd never lose a game!"

Somehow that determination was contagious. When Wendy was around, everyone tried a little harder. He had a way of bringing out the very best in others. The intense purpose in his hazel eyes always made others aware of the principles he stood for, not so much by what he said or did, as by what he was.

But there were times when he admittedly "blew it."

Kent managed to create endless amusement by recounting, to anyone who would listen, one occasion on which Wendy not only brought out the "best" in another student, but demanded it!

Actually, he learned about the incident from Wendy's Mom. One afternoon after school, Wendy admitted to her, "Mom, I really blew it today. I lost my temper completely."

"It happens to all of us Wendy, one time or another. Even Christ was angry with the money changers in the Temple. What happened today?"

"Well, when I came into the locker room from practice, feeling hot and exhausted, one of the team managers was just sitting on the desk. So, I asked him to hand me a towel while I was taking off my helmet. He cursed and told me to get it myself. Well, before I knew it, I had knocked him off the desk. Then I realized what I'd done, so I picked him up and told him never to say that to me again."

"What did he do then?" Jo asked.

"He sort of whispered, 'What was it you wanted, Wendy?'"

Winning was important to Wendy. His ninth grade year at Long Junior High had been a great year. The Buccaneers had won every game and were awarded the district championship. They got used to winning!

Therefore, Wendy's sophomore year at Skyline was something of a shock. It brought him rapidly back to reality! But he accepted the poor season as a learning experience and worked even harder. He considered it a preparation for things to come. Now as a Junior, he was convinced that this was going to be the year.

He believed, as always, in giving one hundred percent, and was sometimes impatient with those who didn't. It was as if he was in a hurry to succeed at everything, demanding more and more of himself and of those around him.

This "urgency" was to become the only cause of serious disagreement between Wendy and Kent. Their Junior year was filled with frustration for both of them. The team wasn't doing well. Even Wendy's enthusiasm and drive didn't manage to instill the determination necessary to create that spark which often makes the difference between winning and losing.

Kent, as quarterback, felt the brunt of the responsibility for pulling the team together.

The more discouraged Kent became, the more Wendy's attempts at motivation depressed him. At last he could stand the pressure no longer and exploded, "Wendy, I am *not* you! I can't give a hundred and twenty percent of myself out there and apparently not many of the others can either. As for me, I give up! I quit! Let someone else call the shots for a while."

"Kent, wait! You can't just walk away. We need you."

"I can't do it, Wendy. I just can't."

For the next three weeks, Kent was a team manager, carrying water bottles and equipment on and off the field, and carefully avoiding Wendy. They lost three straight games. Finally, the team got together to discuss how to bring themselves around. They talked of teamwork and spirit; they took a vote and asked Kent to come back. He still refused, insisting they were better off without him.

On Thursday, the coach sat them all down in the locker room.

"Okay, guys. So, we've lost a few. That's not really what counts. Football is only a game. What makes it so real and important is that it's so much like life. The things we face out there on the field are the same challenges we face in life. There are obstacles, setbacks, risks—we make two yards, then lose six—we win some and get smeared on others. What counts is that we get up and keep on trying!

"No matter what anybody tries to tell you, it's not how many points you chalk up, or how many times you fail, it's how you handle it either way, and what you learn from it. Remember last week against Garland when we had a fourth-and-two on our own forty? I told you to '*Go* for it! It's worth the risk!' That's what I'm telling you today. We're halfway through this season, but giving up will get us nothing! Win or lose, let's go for it—with all we've got!"

There was complete silence in the locker room. Kent was staring down at the floor. He was thinking how often he had tried to run away, to avoid his problems. The Coach was right. And now, he had to make a choice.

The silence was broken when somebody coughed. Kent looked up and all eyes were on him. A familiar grin creased his face; he shrugged and said, "Okay! Let's go for it!"

The remainder of the season showed a steady improvement for the Raiders. They began to operate as a team, and Kent's passing and Wendy's enthusiasm once again inspired them. They soon began to play with a new confidence and maturity, and while the Coach was tougher than ever, inside he was very proud of what they had overcome.

During a break in the school schedule, Wendy's Dad had to make a business trip up the East Coast and decided to take the whole family along. Kent was invited to go too. It was the boys' first look at New England and brief as it was, they managed to cover a lot of territory.

The noisy excitement of New York City amazed them, but didn't impress them as much as crab-fishing in the Atlantic.

The highlight of the whirlwind trip for Wendy was Washington, D.C. The first thing he wanted to see was the Smithsonian Institution.

"Wow, Andy! Look at the tremendous size of those missiles. How do they ever get off the ground?"

"It takes an awful lot of power for a lift-off," Kent said. "I don't think I'd care to be aboard one when it goes."

"Oh, I would!" Wendy's eyes sparkled with excitement.

"Me, too," Andy agreed quickly.

Wendy stood entranced beside the display, lost in his own faraway dreams.

"Come on. There's an aircraft museum inside, we've got to see," Andy urged his brother.

Later, they visited Arlington Cemetery. The awesome sight of the thousands of graves of men who died in the defense of their country left the three boys in a somber mood.

"It makes you feel kind of humble, doesn't it?" Andy said.

"Yeah. And proud," Kent added. "When I look at all those names I wonder if anyone remembers who they were and why they died."

They stood a long while in silent salute, their gaze following the endless rows of white crosses up and down the hillside, across to the resting place of President John F. Kennedy, and so many other Americans who helped to build their nation and fought to keep it free.

There was a small chapel. Wendy noticed a bronze plaque and pointed it out to the others. He read the words aloud:

> *"Living, if it is to be worthy of the name, should mean something more than how many years our hearts beat. The length of our lives, or of living, should be measured in happiness, in what we mean to others."*

"Isn't that beautiful?" Wendy went on. "We should always remember that!"

Kent felt a growing sense of loss as he listened to Wendy's voice, as if the pain and grief from each grave was reaching up to him. The feeling stayed with him a long while, through the rest of their tour. How could he understand death, when he wasn't even sure what life was all about?

The boys treasured many memories from that trip, but none more than those solemn moments at Arlington.

Back home, Kent found it hard to settle into a routine at school. The pressures of competition and schoolwork weighed heavily on him, while Wendy seemed to thrive under their tough schedule. Also, the girls were beginning to feel neglected. Wendy noticed that Amy, in particular, had not been herself recently, but assumed it was because they had had so little time together. So, both of the guys made an effort to squeeze as much fun into the weekends as possible.

They took the girls to hear Sammy Davis, Jr. at the Music Hall and came away breathless from his performance. They went to Lion Country Safari and laughed with delight as the baboons attempted to carry their car away.

It was a big occasion when the Harlem Globe Trotters appeared in Dallas. The girls sat totally captivated by the skillful antics of the players while the boys assured them that it was purely a matter of practice and timing—anyone could do it!

Amy smiled, but her eyes grew suddenly serious and full of honest admiration. "I'm sure you could do anything in the world you really wanted to, Wendy."

For a long moment he looked at her, searching her face for a clue, "What's wrong, Amy?" he asked at last.

Her eyes filled quickly with tears. "It's nothing, Wendy. Just me. I'm too sentimental. Don't worry, though, I'll be just fine."

Wendy took her hand and squeezed it gently. He realized how much they needed to talk. But not now, not here.

The opportunity didn't come until almost a week later. Several times Wendy had planned for a few minutes alone only to be interrupted before he could pin Amy down. She seemed to be avoiding any serious conversation.

On Saturday Wendy and Kent, along with two other friends and their dates, went to the Six Flags Over Texas Amusement Park. It was one of the last few weekends left before the park closed for the season, and there were record crowds to enjoy it. The day had turned surprisingly warm and standing in the long, boisterous lines for the Logride, the excitement and the temperature began to soar.

When their turn came at last, the cool drenching water splashing over into their log canoe came as a welcome relief. The anticipation began to grow unbearable as the boats were pulled higher and higher up the water-filled trough, only to plunge suddenly headlong down the other side. Squealing and laughing, they emerged at last, drenched, but delighted.

The energetic group of teenagers loved every one of the rides in the park. By lunchtime they were all starved, but that was the only thing they could agree on. Kent and Carol voted for pizza, Karen and Steve wanted hamburgers. Everyone had a different choice. Wendy seized the opportunity, determined to make the most of it. He took Amy firmly by the arm and announced, "Everyone for themselves. Let's take off and meet back here at two o'clock." They all seemed to approve the idea and the four couples disappeared, each in a different direction.

Wendy guided Amy through the crowds to the Southern Plantation, a fried chicken restaurant with pretty outdoor tables under a lattice canopy. He picked a quiet corner table overlooking the lagoon. Far below them they could watch an occasional boat sail by and throw crumbs of bread down to the already plump pigeons.

They sat munching the cold chicken and greasy french fries and talked of unimportant things. Only when they'd finished eating, did Wendy ask the question that had been in his thoughts all day. "Amy, have I done something? I know you've been upset lately. Please tell me what's wrong."

"No, it's nothing you've done, Wendy! It's me!" The words began to tumble out in an explosive torrent. "I like you . . . a lot . . . and I love being with you. But I really don't even know who I am yet. My feelings get all confused sometimes. I know it sounds like I'm just jealous—and maybe I am—but I feel like I'm giving one hundred percent to our relationship and you're just "squeezing me in" somewhere between football, school, and motorcycles! I mean, you have such definite plans and dreams. There's just no room in your life for me . . ."

"Amy," Wendy interrupted, "you're more important to me than football, or any plans in the world. Don't you know that?" He reached across the checkered tablecloth and took both her small hands in his own, pressing them tightly, sending tiny ripples of warm excitement through her. "All those dreams are just wishes, but you're here right now. And I need you. I wouldn't hurt you for anything. Amy, I love you!"

Amy felt the tears suddenly hot against her cheeks and tried to blink them away, struggling desperately to maintain her control. There was so much she wanted to say but her throat was constricted by some invisible force which threatened to cut off her air and squeeze all her emotions out through her tear ducts.

"Oh, Wendy," she managed with a gasp, "I've wanted to hear you say that for so long. I . . . I love you, too."

The tears were streaming down her cheeks now for she was powerless to stop the flood of emotion which had been building for so long within her.

Wendy let go of her hands and looked around helplessly for some way to comfort her. People were beginning to stare. Awkwardly he handed her a paper napkin. It seemed a ridiculous situation to Wendy as he sat there feeling miserably responsible for the unhappiness of this girl he loved, and there she sat dabbing futilely at her eyes with a napkin stamped with the picture of a chicken wearing an apron.

"Come on," he urged, taking her hand again. "Let's walk down by the lagoon."

There were fewer people there along the path which curved around an artificial pond. They found a bench beside a cluster of redbud trees and sat down. Wendy was quiet, holding her hand, patiently giving her time to regain her composure. He looked around trying to think what he could say to reassure her. Yet, he was afraid too, of making any commitments he might not be able to live up to.

He found himself in a dilemma. He did love Amy, that much was true. But then, they were only sixteen years old! They were just learning what love is all about, and he certainly wasn't ready to make any promises—even to himself! There were too many uncertainties in their future. No, he had to be careful not to mislead Amy in any way.

But how could he make her understand all that? Suddenly he found himself wishing desperately that he could talk to Kent. Kent would know just what to say.

The long limbs of the redbud trees beside them stretched out over the water, their heart-shaped leaves casting millions of tiny valentine shadows across the water. He reached for a pebble and tossed it into the pool. The hearts blurred into shimmering ringlets that grew larger and larger until they became miniature waves pounding against the painted blue edges of the concrete pond.

At last he spoke, choosing his words carefully. "Amy, we're both pretty young. And we've got a lot of years ahead of us."

She nodded her head in agreement, still unable to find her voice. It was as if all the pent-up emotions finally released had left her drained and empty.

"Whatever is ahead for us," Wendy went on, "we'll face it together. I'll try to consider your feelings more, if you'll agree to understand and not feel left out when there are things I have to do."

"I will, Wendy. I'm sorry for putting you through this . . . but . . . I was so afraid. I really thought you . . . you didn't care. Now that I know how you feel, I promise I . . ."

He put his fingers to her lips to stop her. "Shhh! You don't have to promise anything. From now on, you and I have an understanding. You're my best friend! And friends can count on each other; they don't need promises. No matter what happens tomorrow, we can handle it as long as we can face it honestly and we each care enough to understand how the other one feels."

"Oh, Wendy, thank you for understanding me today. I won't be afraid as long as you're close to me."

He leaned down and kissed her cheek still damp with tears, then gently kissed her lips. She felt all fresh and new inside as if her fears had washed away with her tears and Wendy's words had filled her instead with joy and happiness. His kiss, tender against her face, was like the delicate touch of a butterfly's wings lifting her and freeing her from herself.

"Wendy," she said smiling, "before we go back to join the others, could we pray together?"

"I think that would be perfect," he agreed.

If anyone happened to pass by that way, and noticed the two young people holding hands on the stone bench, their heads bowed, they might have thought it rather odd, but Wendy and Amy wouldn't have minded at all.

"Dear Lord," Amy prayed, "thank you for Wendy. Thank you for what he means to me. Help me to be more understanding, to think less of myself and more about others. Help me to be a better person and a better Christian."

Wendy added, "Dear Father, thank you for loving us and for bringing us together. Help us both to depend on You more and to accept Your will for our lives. Give us the courage to do whatever You ask, and to follow wherever You lead, for we know You will be with us always."

By the time they finally made it back to the agreed-upon meeting place, the others were ready to organize a search party. However, one look at Wendy's beaming smile and Amy's starry eyes, and all their worry was replaced by questions: "What happened?" "What planet did you two visit?" "What'd you do, get lost?"

Wendy held up his hands. "Hey, wait a minute! Let's just say," he paused to wink at Amy, "we found our way back, and everything's great!"

The others applauded loudly and immediately led the way toward the "Mine Train."

It was a perfectly glorious afternoon!

Between the last few football games of the season, and dates with the girls, there was little time for studying; and it suddenly began to show in Kent's grades. Wendy spent many evenings helping him go over American History. Kent couldn't understand how his friend could enjoy learning all that "ancient junk."

Maybe part of Wendy's enthusiasm had to do with a girl in his history class. Minnie. Oh, she wasn't really competition for Amy, but Wendy liked her right away and they quickly became friends.

For Minnie, though, it was a real crush. She was "hooked" the very first day in class as she stared at him sitting across the aisle. His blond hair was neatly combed. He was wearing a blue plaid shirt tucked into the waist of his navy slacks. "I just couldn't believe he was for real," she later told a girlfriend. "He was polite and neat and good-looking too!"

Although Wendy noticed Minnie as well, he was too shy to speak first. So, it was Minnie who finally broke the ice. "I noticed your athletic bag under the desk. Do you play football?"

"Yes, I do," Wendy answered.

"On the J-V team?" Minnie asked, thinking he was too small for the first string.

"No," Wendy said smiling. "On the Varsity."

"Oh, I . . . I see," she gulped and quickly looked away. She tried to appear casually absorbed in the chapter they were supposed to be reading.

After class, it was Wendy who put her at ease. He introduced himself and started right off talking about history, ignoring her earlier remark. If it bothered him, he never admitted it.

Each day Minnie could hardly wait for fifth period to arrive. When she was stumped on a question, Wendy always knew the answer. (And, sometimes when she wasn't really stumped, it was fun to ask him anyway.)

He was always patient with her. He really seemed to enjoy helping her, and the class was free to discuss the lesson. In fact, they often divided into groups to go over chapters together. Minnie always managed to be included in Wendy's group. She even appeared in the lunchroom on occasion with some request or other to make of him.

It was an early November day when the history class was interrupted by the principal's solemn voice over the public address system.

"I am very sorry to inform you of the loss of one of our students. Sally Ross was killed early this morning in a car accident. A memorial service will be held on Thursday."

Minnie's face went white as chalk when the name of her best friend was spoken. Her pencil slipped from her hand and clattered to the floor. Wendy reached out thinking she might fall, but instead, she sprang out of her chair and ran from the room.

A few minutes later when the bell rang, Wendy gathered Minnie's books, retrieved the pencil and walked into the crowded hallway to look for her.

He spotted her, at last, standing far down at the end of the hall by the window. She was staring blindly at the grayness outside. It was a windy, fall day, still warm, yet her arm was cold as ice when he touched her.

"Minnie, I'm very sorry."

"She was my friend, Wendy. I loved her. Oh, God! How could it happen?"

His eyes were bright with emotion but his voice was strong and reassuring as he spoke, "I know how you feel. Don't you wish He would take you instead? But it's up to Him, isn't it? We can't always understand His reasons. But, He loves you and, if you trust Him, it *will* be all right. You'll see."

Minnie could feel the tears now, warm and welcome on her face. "Thanks, Wendy. I'll be okay."

She took her books from his arms and walked away.

That evening Wendy sat on Amy's front porch and told her about his talk with Minnie. "She was so shocked and hurt. I didn't know what to say to her."

"I'm sure whatever you said was a help to her. She's had a lot of problems hasn't she? And this on top."

"Yes. Her Mother and Dad are divorced. She has to help look after her brothers and sisters. I think her mother is very strict, too."

"She has quite a crush on you, you know."

"Aw, I don't think so. She's just a friend. Say! Are you jealous?"

"No, of course not . . . well, maybe just a little. But I think I've learned my lesson, and I don't intend to let anything like that come between us again."

Wendy laughed and kissed her. They sat for a long time, holding hands, watching the clouds move silently across the sky, casting ever-darkening shadows against the moon's brightness. The night was calm and quiet, but inside, they each felt a stirring uneasiness after the events of the day, and even a little guilty about the happiness they shared while others had such sorrow.

6.

Kent stared at the photograph of Wendy standing in the Colorado snow. He remembered the day he had taken it. It was Christmas Eve and they had climbed a mountain together. He even remembered Wendy's words as they climbed, "Heaven must be like this, looking down and seeing the world go on as usual, and yet, none of it very important anymore because of the beauty and peace, and because of the nearness of God . . . Come on, Kent, let's go! I can't wait to see how it feels at the very top!"

They seldom had time to sit and watch television, especially a three-hour show. But Wendy and Amy did watch "Love Story," which was scheduled that week. Amy cried through most of it. Wendy didn't tease her about it, though. In fact, he was surprisingly unimpressed with the picture.

They went out for a hamburger and talked about the sadness of the picture, a romantic tale of true love tragically interrupted by an early death.

"Wendy, it was so sad. How could you keep from crying?" Amy asked.

"Well, I guess I don't look at death like that. I mean, sure it's sad to lose someone, but it shouldn't be like that. They acted as if it is hopeless! Christians look at death as a new beginning. If you *really* believe that Jesus Christ is alive today, then there is nothing hopeless at all about death."

"But aren't you a little bit afraid anyway?"

"That's a hard question to answer," Wendy said honestly, "but, no. I don't think I am. Once when we were flying to Colorado, our plane went through some heavy turbulence. It only lasted a few minutes, but I was scared, at first. Then, all of a sudden, I felt very calm. This feeling of total peace came over me. I've never felt quite so relaxed before in my life. Somehow I knew there was nothing to worry about, everything was taken care of . . . I've thought about it a lot since then.

"I'm beginning to realize that the only things I should worry about are the things I can control. I worry about doing my best, or helping someone else, but I don't waste any time worrying about something that is in God's hands, not mine. I just leave all that up to Him."

"I know that's what we *should* do," Amy said, "but it's not easy. What if you lost someone who was very close to you? Wouldn't you be sad then?"

"Sure. Look, I don't mean to sound like I have all the answers or anything, 'cause I don't. But I do believe that love is stronger than death, and death only exists in this world. I think that's what Jesus meant when He said, 'Be of good cheer, for I have overcome the world.' When we are joined together with Christ, nothing can really separate us—not even death."

"It's only human to want to go on living, Wendy. This life is all we really know about."

"I agree with what Paul said in Philippians, 'For, to me, living means opportunities for Christ, and dying—well, that's better yet!' It's always harder, though, on those who are left behind. We *should* be happy for the one who's gone on. It should be like—like seeing someone off on a long trip. We should say 'Bon Voyage,' or 'See you soon!' But I guess we're too human to do that. So, we hurt and we miss them terribly. But deep inside, we're still okay, because we know that they are in heaven and that we'll be joining them soon. That's the difference between what death means to Christians and the kind of false sadness in the picture."

"I know you're right, but it was still a good movie!" Amy insisted. "I'm sorry. I guess I just love a sentimental story."

Wendy laughed, "I thought love meant 'never having to say you're sorry.' "

December 22nd was Wendy's birthday. So Amy took *him* out to dinner. They went to the Spaghetti Warehouse, one of their favorite places, and spent a leisurely two hours eating and talking. Amy seemed especially talkative that night, Wendy thought. He was finished long before she was.

"How's your spaghetti?" he asked finally.

"Oh, it's delicious. I'm enjoying every bite."

Wendy glanced at his watch. "If we're going to the concert maybe you could eat just a little faster?"

"What time is it?"

"It's nearly eight."

"Oh, good," Amy looked relieved. "I mean, I'm really so full, I couldn't eat another bite anyway."

As Wendy helped her with her coat, she turned anxiously, "Oh, Wendy, I must have left the envelope with the tickets at your house. I'm sorry, but could we please stop and get them?"

Wendy looked a bit perturbed but, always the gentleman, he only said, "Sure," and glanced anxiously at his watch again.

Amy chattered all the way back to the house, while Wendy began to feel more and more irritable as the hands on his watch moved on past eight.

At last he slowed to a stop in front of the house and started to get out. "I'll run in and get it. You can just wait here." But his words were lost, for Amy was already out of the car.

"I'm not sure where I left it, Wendy. You may have trouble finding it."

"Oh, for pete's sake," Wendy mumbled under his breath. He sighed deeply, and escorted her to the front door. The house was dark, as his parents were away for the evening. He fumbled with the lock and finally opened the door.

Wendy stepped inside first and reached for the light switch. Suddenly every light in the room came on at once. He blinked his eyes in surprise as a dozen kids in assorted shapes and sizes yelled, "Happy Birthday!"

Wendy couldn't believe it. "How did you ever do this without letting me know?"

"Kent planned the whole thing," someone shouted.

"Aw, it was Amy's idea," Kent offered.

"Amy!" Wendy exclaimed. "You should have seen her eating in slow motion. I've never seen anyone eat spaghetti, one piece at a time! Now I see why."

Amy laughed with relief. "I was so afraid you wouldn't agree to come by here. And that two hours seemed like an eternity!"

Everyone joined in when Mike started singing "Happy Birthday" and Karen came through the door from the dining room with a huge cake ablaze with seventeen candles.

When everyone was eating, and Kent was on his third slice, Wendy spoke very seriously for a moment, "Hey, everybody. I want you all to know how much I appreciate your doing this. You're the greatest!"

Kent stood up solemnly, holding out a glass of Dr. Pepper, "No, Wendy. *You're* the greatest . . . for a shy clown, that is!"

After a round of applause, they all raised their glasses as a toast, "To Bozo!" they shouted. Wendy blushed, which only encouraged the frivolity, until Amy and Carol saved him by bringing in an armload of gaily wrapped packages.

"Aw, gosh," Wendy murmured. "You guys shouldn't have done that."

"You better see what's inside," someone advised, "before you pass judgment."

He opened package after package of "gag" gifts. The last one he opened was a pair of socks, one brown and one blue!

Later when the others had left, Amy and Carol attacked the last of the cleanup detail in the kitchen, while Kent and Wendy picked up in the living room.

"It was a terrific party, Kent," Wendy said. "I don't know how to thank you."

"Oh, Wendy, it was a blast! I didn't do anything anyway; the girls did all the work!"

"Well, it's really neat to have so many good friends. I'm a very lucky person. Sometimes I feel like I have just everything—things I really don't deserve."

"Why on earth would you say that, Wendy? You're the best person I know!"

"No, Kent. Not really. Inside, I'm not good at all. I keep promising myself that I'll do better, that I won't lose my temper, that I'll be more patient. It's just that I'm so anxious for things to happen, and it irritates me when people don't do what they tell you they will. I've really prayed a lot about it.

"I've even started writing little notes and putting them in conspicuous places to remind myself to be more patient." Wendy went on, "If I didn't know that God loves me in spite of all my faults, I don't know what I'd do."

For once, Kent was speechless. He couldn't think of anything he could say at that moment to console his friend. Much later, he thought of so many reassuring things he *wished* he'd said. But somehow he'd been stunned by Wendy's mood. It was as if he'd never realized before that Wendy got discouraged too.

And if Wendy, who was so good, recognized and admitted out loud his need for God, then how much more did Kent himself need Him! Kent—who was so stubborn and independent, who was convinced he didn't need anyone but himself—was there even a slight possibility that he might be wrong?

That was one possibility he was not yet prepared to face!

Wendy's Mom and Dad had a real surprise in store as a birthday *and* Christmas gift . . . A skiing trip to Colorado. Kent and Amy, and Andy's friend, David, were all invited. Kent and David accepted, but Amy declined because her grandparents were coming to spend Christmas with her family.

The slopes were glistening with thick blankets of snow and smoothly inviting as Wendy and Kent took them on in eager anticipation. The wind deposited frosty crystals of white on their faces while they raced their way from the high crest to the valley below, hearts pounding with the thrill of speed and the freedom of motion.

Kent reached the bottom first, glided to a stop and looked back at Wendy pushing to catch up. He watched horrified as Wendy missed the last curve, his skis flying straight out from under him while he turned a perfect backward flip, landing in an awkward heap at the foot of the hill. Kent hurried over to him as fast as his clumsy skis would allow.

"Are you hurt?"

"Naw, I'm fine. That was close though, wasn't it? I *almost* landed on my feet!"

Kent breathed a sigh of relief, "Wendy, you're an absolute nut!"

The next morning there was four inches of fresh snow on the slopes, accompanied by a gusty wind.

"Hey, Kent, let's go mountain climbing. We can rent a sled and go all the way to the top!"

"I might have known you'd say that. Nothing halfway for Wendy. It's the top or nothing."

So, off they went, bundled up against the cold, trudging up an impossibly tall mountain in snow so deep it covered their boots. Pulling the sleds behind them at least insured an easier way down.

They climbed steadily for over an hour before stopping to rest. The deep snow and high altitude made breathing difficult, and their muscles began to ache with weariness.

"It's so quiet and still up here. Almost as if the whole world were asleep under a quilt of snow."

Wendy, still catching his breath, nodded in agreement.

They were quiet for a while absorbing the peacefulness. Then Wendy spoke, his voice soft in the stillness, "I think I'd like to stay up here for a long time, just watching. Heaven must be like this, looking down and seeing the world go on as usual, and yet, none of it very important anymore because of the beauty and peace, and because of the nearness of God. Come on, Kent, let's go! I can't wait to see how it feels at the very top!"

"Oh, boy! If I make it, I'll be too tired to feel anything!" Later, Kent remembered how amazed he'd been at Wendy's determination and stamina. He had felt exhausted and ready to call it quits and start back, but not Wendy! Wendy was ready to go on, always ready to accept a new challenge.

So, on they trudged, their boots thudding in the soft snow, leaving deep-pocketed trails behind. Several times Kent wanted to quit, but there was no stopping Wendy. Even though they began to feel as if their lungs would burst, they plunged onward and upward, their goal growing ever nearer.

At last they were there! A tremendous surge of emotion engulfed them and they both fell gasping onto the soft blanket of snow. They were elated, thrilled with a sense of their own accomplishment, and yet, awed at the solitude and almost reverent tranquility about them. Wendy was right. Though they didn't say much, they both felt the atmosphere of isolation from the world below and the overwhelming power of God who in His great love, allows such precious moments of awareness.

They stayed at the summit for a while, absorbing the still loveliness. Then they began the reckless descent, using the sleds wherever the landscape permitted.

Two-thirds of the way down, they climbed onto the sleds for the last long winding slope. After several unscheduled turns, Kent somehow managed to wind up on his back in the snow. His sled, having a mind of its own, easily beat him to the bottom. Seeing Wendy sail by laughing heartily at his predicament didn't especially help his frame of mind.

By the time he reached the bottom, he could still hear the strange sounds of muffled giggles as Wendy pretended to check his sled. But Kent had prepared his own counter measure. The huge snowball caught Wendy square in the back. He turned quickly in hot pursuit as Kent took off—trudging awkwardly through the deep snow.

Kent was laughing now, but as he glanced back at the lengthening distance between them, the expression on Wendy's face was startlingly serious. He wasn't laughing, or even smiling. He was only determined. Somehow, the look in his eyes revealed how important it was to him to win.

Kent remembered other races and suddenly, for no reason he could understand, this one became important to him, too. In a brief moment all these thoughts rushed through his mind as he unconsciously changed his pace. In another minute Wendy had caught him and smothered him with snow.

The moment dissolved into laughter. But long afterwards, Kent remembered that look of urgency and was glad that Wendy had won.

That night there was a Christmas party for all the guests at the hotel. The boys lounged beside the huge stone fireplace, open on all four sides. They met some girls from Georgia and spent the evening talking, and playing chess and backgammon. There was all the hot apple cider and popcorn they could eat and drink.

At eleven o'clock there was a movie scheduled in the dining room, but the Hickmans had their own idea of how to celebrate Christmas Eve. Just before midnight, as arranged, they all met in Bob and Jo's room to exchange the small gifts they had brought along, tucked carefully away in their suitcases.

Andy was elected to read the Christmas story from the second chapter of Luke. Bob and Kent collapsed in the two easy chairs. Jo sat perched, with one leg underneath her, on the huge yellow-quilted king-size bed. Wendy and David sprawled on the floor, Wendy on one elbow, and David on his stomach, resting his chin on his hands. All of them listened quietly, absorbed in the story of events which had occurred almost two thousand years before, yet changed not only their lives, but the course of the entire world.

Wendy said very little that evening. Kent supposed he was thinking of Amy so far away. When they were back in their room alone, and had fallen exhausted into their beds and turned out the light, Wendy spoke earnestly in the darkness, "Kent, there's something I've been wanting to tell you."

"Um . . ." Kent groaned sleepily. "If you're going to tell me there's really no Santa Claus, I don't want to hear it!"

"Be serious, Kent. I just want you to know how much I appreciate your friendship. I know sometimes I get carried away with my enthusiasm and I . . . I just thought you ought to know . . . you're the very best friend anybody ever had."

Kent was suddenly wide awake. "Wendy, I don't know what to say. You're . . ."

"You don't need to say anything, Kent. I just really wanted you to know how I feel."

"You're okay too, Bozo. For a shy clown!" Kent said, disguising his embarrassment. He was still awake a long while later, painfully aware of how much Wendy meant to him, both as a friend and as a Christian example.

On Christmas morning the world outside was a crystal white wonderland. During the night another layer of soft snow had fallen leaving no trace of all the hard-packed footprints of the day before. Diamonds of ice glistened in the bright sunlight illuminating a fresh and glorious new world breathlessly awaiting the arrival of the first bold explorers.

Wendy and Kent, Andy and David rented a couple of sleds and struck out in search of the perfect hill. They soon discovered the ideal spot for a downhill run, a narrow canyon formed between two slopes. A curved and twisting road led through the canyon and up the mountain toward an old, seldom-used ski slope.

Dragging the sleds uphill was hard work in the deep snow, but when they climbed on, two to each sled, for the downhill trip, it was freestyle fun. Steering the clumsy projectile was about as impossible as trying to squeeze toothpaste into a straw. More often than not, they wound up tumbling into a snowbank and came out resembling giant snowballs with assorted protruding arms and legs.

After a series of major failures, interspersed with minor successes, they began to get the hang of it. "If you'll keep your big feet up on the side boards, Kent, we can balance this thing," Wendy insisted.

"I'm trying to! Your legs keep pushing them off. Can't you pull them in closer?"

"Closer! You're taking up two-thirds of the room now, I might as well be riding on a ski!"

"You probably couldn't steer that either," Kent mumbled under his breath as he gave the sled a sudden shove.

Wendy was struggling to untangle his pant leg from under Kent's heavy boot, and was totally unprepared for the surprise start. The unexpected jerk threw him off balance. Kent reached out to keep his companion from falling sideways and the whole sled tipped over, tumbling both its passengers into the snow and sending them rolling head over heels down the hill. It was a long roll to the bottom. Luckily the sled missed landing on top of them.

They ended up buried in a four-foot snowdrift. Andy and David hurried over to see if they were hurt. Like two grizzly bears coming out of hibernation, Kent and Wendy, growling and snorting, dug their way out and stood up shaking and sputtering. Then, exactly at the same instant, each one pointed at the other and yelled, "You clumsy idiot!"

They both froze, each staring at the other, while the echo of their voices in unison bounced off the canyon walls, "You clumsy idiot! idiot!! idiot!! idiot!!"

Andy and David broke into fits of laughter and were soon joined by the two "clumsy idiots." Wendy gave Kent a friendly bear hug and they scrambled through the snowdrift together to retrieve the errant sled.

7.

The sharp echo of Wendy's words came back to him, "Someday, Kent, you're going to find you can't handle it alone . . . And then you'll know what it is to let go completely, to put everything in His hands, and trust Him with all of it!"

It was tough settling down to school again after the holidays. The boys looked forward to weekends more than ever.

January 16th was Superbowl Sunday! The Hickmans planned a big day with Bob's brother, Johnny, and his family joining them to watch the game. Johnny's children, Linda, Jay, and Karen, had practically grown up with Wendy and Andy. The two families had shared many camping and vacation trips, as well as holidays together.

Johnny's wife, Joanna, was always a great cook and had brought a scrumptious coconut cake which didn't last through halftime.

After the game, the boys played pool while the girls helped with the cleanup in the kitchen. Then Wendy and Jay took off their shirts to show Andy a few wrestling holds. Although the two boys were about the same size, Jay was a year older and a member of the wrestling team at his school.

Yet even with Jay's added skill, Wendy was the stronger of the two, his muscles well-toned from Coach Miles' strenuous off-season, weight training program.

They circled each other warily, bare arms smacking loudly as each tried to grasp the other in an armhold. In one quick movement, Jay wrapped a leg around Wendy's knee, pulling him off balance with a shoulder grip, and they both tumbled to the floor in a jumble of writhing muscles accompanied by appropriate grunts and groans.

Jay was the first to swallow his pride and yell, "Calf-rope!"

Wendy's confidence began to surge. "Hey, Andy," he called, "watch this one." He lunged at Jay, intending to wrap him in a bear hug, but this time, Jay twisted away, grabbed Wendy's arm, and skillfully turned it under with a forearm lock. It was Wendy's turn to yell "Calf-rope."

The horseplay continued for a while until Wendy's Mom decided the furniture was in danger, and ended the contest.

"That weight lifting is really paying off, Wen. You're in better shape than I am," Jay admitted.

"Coach Miles really puts us through it. And Dad keeps me on a heavy training diet too—malts with raw eggs, lots of protein, very little sugar, and no soft drinks. Mom pours down the vitamins." Wendy flexed his muscles and expanded his chest fully. With a W. C. Fields drawl, he quipped, "You're looking at one of the healthiest specimens of the space age!"

"Yeah," Andy agreed quickly, "only all the 'space' is in his head!"

Monday was the hardest day of all to face football off-season workouts. Kent struggled with his gear, already feeling tired and hot. "Wow! This is for the birds! Hey, Wendy, why don't we take up somethin' easier, like golf?"

Wendy didn't laugh.

"Hey, you don't look so good. Are you okay?"

"Sure. I'm just a little tired, I guess."

"Maybe you should tell the coach, and not work out today."

"Naw, I'm okay. We've got a lot of work to do before next season."

Kent didn't argue. He knew Wendy wouldn't quit for anything. They went out together to warm up.

They ran a couple of laps, did some pushups and then started down the prearranged course, stepping through tires placed side by side in long rows.

The coach's voice rang in their ears as he urged them to, "Move it! Move it! Get those knees up higher!"

Kent pushed ahead at a steady pace like a machine, functioning without feeling or thought. He reached the end of the track and turned automatically to follow the course, when suddenly, the scene before him sent a chill of alarm through him. His perspiration quickly dissolved into an icy shiver.

Down the field a group of the boys had stopped and were standing helplessly by as the coaches worked frantically over a fallen form. As Kent reached them, they were putting an oxygen cup over Wendy's mouth. They tried external heart massage and mouth-to-mouth resuscitation, but it was no use.

Wendy was gone.

The boys all stood riveted as the ambulance arrived and quickly left again with its lifeless passenger, the siren piercing sharply through the numbness of their senses. Silently their eyes came to rest on the blue and red jersey, crumpled on the ground, the number "45" stamped across it. Tears streamed shamelessly down some of their faces, dropping onto their sweat-soaked shirts.

There was shock, pain, helplessness written on every face. Jake, "the Black Bass," mumbled, "Oh, God! Not Wendy, please not Wendy!" There were rivulets of tears shining on his black cheeks.

The coaches quietly brought them back to reality, urging them gently toward the locker room.

Practice was over.

Kent bent down, lifted the shirt from the ground and held it tightly against him. As he stumbled blindly toward the gym, the pain and numbness turned to rising anger. Why? Oh, God! How? How could You allow this?

When he reached the locker room, he laid the jersey down beside the neat stack of Wendy's clothes, all carefully folded, as if he would be back any minute to put them on again. He just stood there for several long minutes, staring.

Then he yanked his helmet off and threw it as hard as he could. It crashed against the bench and plummeted across the floor into the wall. He turned and slammed his fist hard against his locker door. The force pushed the latch free and the door flew open, clanging loudly against the door beside it.

There, right in front of his eyes, was a yellowed scrap of paper taped to the inside of the door, and Wendy's neatly printed words, "Smile, Kent, God loves you!"

He backed up and sat down heavily on the bench, staring at the note, until the tears came, clouding out his vision and choking him with an invisible weight of grief.

Kent went to the funeral home Tuesday evening. There were several people there standing in small groups, whispering, wiping tears from their faces. He sat down in a green chair with velvet flowered cushions. All he could think of was how Wendy would laugh if he could see him, all dressed up in a monkey suit, sitting on a bunch of silly-looking green velvet flowers.

He got up and moved across the room. Friends came over and shook his hand, patted his shoulder, spoke a few words in sympathy. He didn't hear what they said. He just smiled and nodded.

Amy came in, supported by her mother on one side and Carol on the other. She looked down at Wendy's peaceful face and began to cry hysterically. They helped her out and took her to another room somewhere. Later Carol came back and took his hand. "Kent, could you come and talk to Amy? She's asking for you."

Amy was sitting on a brown sofa as he walked in. She was wearing a light blue dress. It had dark spots on the skirt. He stared at them until slowly it came to him that they were wet spots where her tears had fallen on her lap. He wasn't thinking clearly. Everything was moving in a giant collage of colors, like a dream with no order or sense.

Amy looked up at him. "Oh, Kent," and she began to cry again.

He sat beside her and held her, and they both cried together. The others stepped out and left them alone. In a few minutes she tried to talk. "Kent, I can't believe it. It can't be true. . . . It's just a bad dream, isn't it?"

"I wish it were, Amy."

"We . . . we just talked about dying a few weeks ago." The tears were still streaming down her face. She spoke through her sobs. "He . . . he said that love was stronger than death, and that we should say 'Bon Voyage,' and . . . and, Oh Kent, I can't . . ."

"I know, Amy. It's okay. We'll be okay . . . we'll be okay . . ."

Hundreds of kids came that day to stand quietly in the back of the crowded funeral home. They all loved him. They all knew that a very special part of their lives was gone—yet a more precious gift would always be theirs because he had been their friend.

Tom Collingsworth came from Sky Ranch to help with the service. His words were not the usual ones for a funeral. He did not speak of a faraway heaven, or a reunion one day in the future. He spoke of the present, of victory *now,* of rejoicing in Christ and His triumph over death. He repeated the phrase Wendy had used so often, being "alive in Christ." Kent wasn't sure he understood that completely, but the words had a comforting sound.

Tom read a brief testimony which had been found on Wendy's desk. He had written it for a meeting of the FCA scheduled the following week. Tom's voice was a little shaky as he read the words:

> *"As most of us know, athletics is constantly presenting great challenges to those who participate in the field of sports. Sometimes these challenges become too great for me to handle. I know that this has happened to me many times. The difference between those who lose and those who win over their failures is determined by how the failure affects them personally. I know at times I have asked myself why I was even out for athletics, but I know that athletics holds many rewards for those who play the games.*
>
> *"If I were to name the one thing that prevented me from quitting long ago, it would be the crutch I leaned on when the going got rough. I always had a Friend to talk to about my problems and decisions.*
>
> *"This person I am speaking of is Jesus Christ. He is alive and real to each of us who know Him personally. He can be seen in the faces of those people at Skyline who have decided to follow the Word of God.*
>
> *"I owe all I have done in this lifetime to Christ. To me and others who know Christ, He stands for strength and assurance. I*

> *know without this strength that Christ has given me, I would have given up all hope of ever playing football; and I would have missed something that has taught me much."*

Kent stood with the family at the front of the chapel. There were tears, and sadness too, but also an overwhelming sense of peace on every face. He wondered how they could accept it and speak at the same time of rejoicing? Oh, he understood intellectually that Wendy was alive in heaven. But it was emotionally unacceptable that, in one impossibly swift moment, he could have been physically and irrevocably removed from this earth, and from our sphere of knowledge.

Kent felt so helpless. There was nothing he could do to lessen the pain for himself or anyone else.

At the close of the service, Wendy's friends walked quietly past, many pausing to say, "Thank you for being my friend and for sharing God's love with me."

Hal, Karen, John, James, Carol, Ken, Jay, Billy—so many others. Minnie paused a moment and placed a rose on his hand.

Then the others were gone and only the family remained. Bob asked Kent to stay, "Wendy would have wanted you to," he said.

Kent wasn't sure he could stay. He wanted to run as long and as hard as he could until he dropped with exhaustion. Maybe if he ran fast enough, reality would become blurred and he could forget for a moment.

But he stayed, standing still and quiet, while his heart screamed inside him. He watched the parents of his best friend lean down and kiss his cheek for the last time. In a blur of tears, he heard Bob whisper, "Goodnight, son. We'll see you in the morning."

There was a brief service at Restland Cemetery. Groups of friends gathered with the family to pray and comfort each other. There were tears, but through the tears, triumph glowed undeniably.

Kent held Amy's hand. He did all he could to help, still knowing that their grief could not be shared. They both were to learn that each person must come to his own terms in his own way, with that most painful experience.

Afterwards, he helped her into the car with her parents. Carol and Karen went along to stay with her. Then, Kent walked back alone and stood beside the mound of flowers. Their fragrance drifted across the air with a thick sweetness, leaving a bitter-sweet taste in his mouth. He stood still, his head bowed, his eyes dark and unseeing, while his thoughts rushed frantically in all directions.

His senses still rebelled at the realization that Wendy was gone. And yet, it was there looming ahead of him. Stubbornly he kept hearing Wendy's voice, seeing his smile, wanting to make it all a hideous nightmare. But there before him, the flowers quivered in the chill air, in an unspoken denial of his plea. . . .

And suddenly, Kent was listening to the sharp echo of Wendy's words, "Someday, Kent, you're going to find you can't handle it alone. And then you'll know what it is to let go completely, to put everything in His hands, and trust Him with all of it!"

"Dear God," he prayed aloud, "Wendy was right. I can't handle this alone. I just can't! I'm so afraid! How can I face a world without him? He was always there when I needed him. He always knew how I felt, understood things I couldn't even put in words. How can I accept it? Why did it happen? Why Wendy? Please help me, Lord. Help me to understand!"

Kent stood there blinded by his tears. The flowers still trembled before him. A thin blue ribbon, lifted by a wisp of breeze, pulled free from a spray of roses and slipped unnoticed to the ground.

When at last Kent turned and walked away, the blue ribbon lay pressed against the leaves beneath his foot. The words printed across it in gold lettering read, "The Lord is near to him who calls upon His name" Psalm 145:18.

8

"I asked Wendy once what heaven is like," Andy said. " 'Like winning a race,' he told me. 'When you cross the finish line, everyone comes to welcome you and the angels have a giant parade and celebration in your honor!' "

Kent spent a lot of time during the next few weeks at the Hickman home. He felt a strong need to be near them. He played ball with Andy, and took him skating one Saturday early in March.

They were sitting together on the bench, putting on their skates when Andy suddenly looked up with tears in his eyes. "Wendy and I both got new skates for Christmas. His are still sitting in the corner of his room."

Kent thought of the bedroom Wendy had shared with his brother. Andy's things had been moved into another room and Wendy's door closed for a while. It would take time before they would be ready to put his things away.

"I still can't believe it," Andy was saying. "He won't be using those skates—ever!"

"I know, Andy. I know how much you miss him. It's been hard for all of us. I guess we'll never get used to it."

"All my life, Kent, I've had Wendy to look up to, to count on. Now I feel kind of lost. It's like part of me is missing . . . Did you know we were both baptized at the same time?"

Kent shook his head and Andy went on.

"We used to read our Bibles together at night. Wendy would explain the parts I didn't understand. Once in a while, when he didn't know about something, we'd go and ask Mom. I especially remember when we were real little, we were reading John 14, and Wendy got so excited when he read about Jesus coming back to take us to heaven with Him. I asked him what heaven is like. He thought a minute before he answered. 'Like winning a race,' he said. 'When you cross the finish line, everyone comes to welcome you and the angels have a giant parade and celebration in your honor.' "

Kent couldn't help smiling as he thought of Wendy leading a parade of angels.

Andy smiled too and said, "I guess that beats skating any day!"

They both laughed. Kent put his arm around Andy's shoulder. "You're okay, Andy. You're really okay."

Kent sat many quiet evenings just talking with the Hickman family and friends who dropped by. He put his arms around Jo and they cried together sometimes, and sometimes laughed remembering the happiness and joy Wendy had brought to them.

Bob was a pillar of strength for all of them. He had lost a son, and yet his faith was stronger than ever. Together, they accepted Jesus' own words in Luke 10:20, that we should "Rejoice for our names are written in heaven!"

Kent was amazed to realize that the Hickmans actually offered comfort to all those who came expecting to comfort them.

The next few months were a revelation to Kent as one by one, friends and acquaintances sought him out to tell him how Wendy had touched their lives.

Jake called to him one day after practice. "Hey, wanna help me move some stuff for Coach Miles?"

"Sure," Kent answered.

They talked in spurts as they dragged the heavy equipment back into the storage area.

"You know, I sure do miss Wendy. He used to cheer me up sometimes."

"Yeah. I know what you mean," Kent agreed.

"Just thinking about him makes me feel better," Jake said.

"Really?"

"I always thought that if there was a God, He was too busy running the universe to worry about me and my little problems. Wendy told me once that we never recognize what God gives us until He takes it away. Now, for the first time, I'm beginning to see what he meant. At first I couldn't believe that a good God would take away someone like Wendy. But then, when I think of what Wendy was like, I want to get to know his God too. I guess I should thank Him for letting Wendy stay as long as he did."

"He can be *your* God, too, Jake . . . I'd say you've come a long way."

"Yeah, maybe. Thanks to Wendy."

"Yes. And thank God for Wendy!"

One day Kent bumped into Paul Stone, a history teacher from their days at Long Junior High.

He immediately spoke of Wendy. "He was always a leader. We teachers tend to expect more of young people like that. And he never let me down. I noticed that the other students not only shared my respect for him, but looked for his approval as well, and that's a real tribute."

"He had a lot of admiration for you, too, sir," Kent said. "Did you know he had decided to become a teacher?"

"No, I didn't. He would have made a good one. I do know I'm a better teacher for having known him. You see, Wendy restored my faith in humanity and in my profession by reminding me there are still some fine young people in the world. Yes, he would have been a fine teacher."

"In a way," Kent said thoughtfully, "he already was."

There were many others too, whose lives were affected by Wendy's influence. Minnie came to Kent one Thursday in the school lunchroom. "If you have any time today, I'd like to talk to you about something."

"Okay," Kent answered. "How about in the library after school?"

"That's fine. I'll see you there." As she walked away Minnie remembered how often she had gone to the cafeteria on some excuse or other just to see Wendy for a minute.

That afternoon she was already waiting in the library when Kent arrived.

"Hi!" He put his books across from hers and plopped down onto a chair. "I've got a fifteen-page history report due next week and I haven't started yet! You don't happen to have any great notes on the American Revolution, do you?"

Minnie shook her head and held one finger to her lips reminding Kent of the library rules. "Sorry, I'm afraid I'm having trouble myself," she admitted.

"Ah, well," he said in a softer voice, "something will turn up; and if all else fails, there's always Charles!"

Minnie smiled, well aware that Kent was only kidding. Charles, although an "A" student was very fat and unpopular, and often the subject of brutal jokes. Recently there had been a lot of trouble when it was discovered that some members of the football team had bribed Charles to write papers for them by promising to arrange dates for him with one of the cheerleaders.

"What was it you wanted to talk to me about, Minnie? Not history, I hope?"

"No," she said. "I was wondering if you would look at something." She glanced down at her notebook. "I . . . I've written a poem about Wendy. I just wanted to say how much he meant to me and this is the only way I could think of. I hope you won't think I'm crazy or anything."

"Of course not. I'd love to read it, Minnie. You'd be surprised how many people have talked to me about him. Everyone who knew him, even slightly, felt close to him. He touched so many lives. I'm only beginning to learn how many."

"You mentioned Charles," Minnie said. "I guess he's one of those, too."

"Charles?" Kent asked in surprise. "I didn't know they even knew each other."

"Well, I've been talking to him lately. I really feel sorry for him. He mentioned they were friends, and said Wendy treated him differently than anyone else did; that he seemed to respect him as a person. Charles went on about how Wendy had told him he admired him for being an "A" student, and that God looks at what's on the inside of us and that's what counts.

"Charles is going to be okay, I think, Kent."

"I can't get over it!" Kent said in amazement. "I was with Wendy so much of the time. But I didn't realize that he was so special to everyone else too."

Minnie's eyes were filled with tears. "I never believed that anyone could really live a Christian life in today's world without being considered a freak, or a weirdo. But Wendy did live that way, and everyone loved and respected him."

Minnie handed Kent a piece of paper from her notebook, and watched anxiously as he read:

TO WENDY . . .

You made me see right from wrong
and what I now must do,
You brought out a love deep inside,
With Jesus Christ, I will survive.
I never realized how happy I could be,
but it was you, Wendy,
Who brought this out in me.

I thank you now for just being
a part of my life,
But I wish it could have been longer.

Everytime I think of you, I am
happy because I know you are in heaven
With your Creator.
But even though I see you no more,
Your presence is everywhere.
Yes, you have left a part of yourself
behind, with me.
I will carry your memory always.

"It's beautiful, Minnie!"

"Would you give it to his parents for me, Kent? I'd like for them to have it."

"Of course, but why don't you come with me and give it to them yourself? They'd be so glad to see you."

"I don't think I could do that. I've never even met them. I wouldn't know what to say, and I'd probably cry and make them feel worse!"

"Minnie, don't you think *they* understand how you feel? And, just by being there, they'll know you care and that will mean a lot to them."

"Maybe you're right," she agreed.

"Why don't we go right now, before you change your mind?"

Kent tucked the poem into the pocket of her sweater, picked up her books and his own, and started for the door.

"Now?" Minnie had no choice but to follow.

By the time they arrived at the Hickman home, however, Minnie was ready to back out. "Oh, Kent, please! I don't think I can do it."

"Not even for Wendy?"

Jo Hickman answered the door.

"Mrs. Hickman, this is Minnie. Minnie, this is Wendy's Mom," Kent introduced them.

There were suddenly tears in Jo's eyes as she reached out and put her arms around Minnie. Then, Minnie was crying too, and it was good for both of them, a momentary sharing of their grief.

Minnie spoke first, "Mrs. Hickman, Wendy was my friend, and I loved him."

"I know," Jo said smiling. "He loved you, too. He spoke of you many times. Come in and meet Bob and Andy."

They sat and talked a while of less important things: school, football, plans for the future. Later Bob challenged Kent and Andy to a game of pool, and the three of them disappeared into the game room and left Jo and Minnie alone.

Immediately Wendy became the subject of their conversation.

"Wendy told me of some of your family problems, Minnie. He was concerned about you. I think he appreciated his own family a lot more after learning how difficult it has been for you."

"You all meant a great deal to him. He talked about you constantly."

Jo spoke sincerely, "He loved the times the two of you spent in the counseling office together."

"We both volunteered to work there. I only did it because Wendy was going to be there. We used to sort stacks of cards, and it was quiet, and we had long talks about—just *everything*."

Minnie handed Jo the paper from her pocket and waited quietly while she read. When she looked up again and wiped the tears from her dark eyes, Minnie continued, "He helped me in so many ways. He caused me to really look at myself, maybe for the first time and accept what I am—good *and* bad. You know, to me God has always been just a word. But Wendy showed me a real concept of what God is, a loving Father who made us as we are, not a demanding Creator holding a rulebook over our heads. But I still can't understand how He could take Wendy. He was so good and kind. Mrs. Hickman, how can you accept his death?"

"I don't, Minnie," Jo assured her. "I *accept his life!* When you accept Jesus Christ as Saviour and Master of your life, you also accept the abolishment of death. Jesus died in our place to give us *eternal* life. So, you see, Wendy isn't really gone; he exists in a new dimension of his life."

Jo continued, slowly. "It is beyond our comprehension now, Minnie, but I believe with all my heart that one day I will see and understand it all clearly."

"That's like my dream," Minnie exclaimed!

"Tell me about it," Jo suggested.

"A few nights ago, I dreamed that Wendy and I were walking together. He held my hand and led me along a path where there were trees and flowers and people passing by. They all looked so happy and peaceful.

"As we were climbing a hill, Wendy suddenly let go of my hand and waved as he walked on. Somehow I knew I could not go any farther. I called to him, 'Wait! How do I get back?' He pointed toward a huge glass box I hadn't noticed before. As I walked toward it, I could see it was full of people shouting and fighting, and I was suddenly afraid.

"There was a man at the door of the box. He told me to walk through and not to be afraid, that nothing would hurt me. So I started through. The crowds were yelling and pushing, but no one touched me. It was as if I had a protective shield around me. Then, suddenly, I woke up."

"What do you think your dream meant?"

"Well, I guess at first, I wanted to die too. But that decision isn't ours to make. Now, I'm beginning to learn more and more about the power and the love of God, which Wendy talked about. And I know He will guide and protect me until that time comes for me to go."

"Don't make the mistake though, Minnie, of thinking that nothing can hurt you along the way. The devil would like you to believe that; so when he throws problems at you, you'll begin to doubt your faith. God doesn't promise to make things easy. We still must endure pain and sorrow. And when someone we love is taken, we suffer dearly. But God's promise is that He will never leave us alone. His love surrounds and comforts us. His Spirit will guide us through all the troubles of this life and into that new dimension which we call heaven. All we need to do is hold on to His hand and trust Him to keep that promise."

Minnie was sure she would remember everything Wendy's Mom had told her. "I appreciate your listening to me and your advice. If it's all right, I'd like to come to see you again sometime."

"Please do! Anytime you can," Jo assured her.

A few weeks later, Kent spoke with Mrs. Marguerite Smith, another of Wendy's former teachers. She asked about the Hickmans.

"It's been very difficult for them, of course," he told her. "But their strength and faith are amazing."

"I've missed him," Mrs. Smith admitted. "For two years he sat in the third row, fifth chair from the front in my class. And every day as he left carrying his athletic bag, he always stopped to say 'Have a nice day.' He was never too busy to stop, or to help someone else. Almost every day, I noticed other students asking Wendy's help or his opinion. He was never too busy to listen, and he wasn't too busy when the Lord called him." She spoke softly. "I was devastated when I heard of Wendy's death and I prayed for understanding. I couldn't help but ask, 'Dear God, why Wendy?' I felt an answer almost immediately,

'Who was more ready than he?' As much as we all loved him, I believe he was one of the few people I've ever known whom I would consider ready for God's call. Even in his few years on this earth, I believe he left no stone unturned, no word unsaid, no task yet undone in his life."

What an amazing testimony for a seventeen-year-old boy! Kent would never cease to be amazed at the legacy of love which Wendy had left behind.

It was months before Kent and Amy talked about Wendy. Time had only begun to slowly heal the hurt which burned so deeply in her eyes, that faraway, guarded look which haunted Kent. At first, she wouldn't let anyone be close to her, as if she feared any attachment. And no one dared to mention Wendy's name. She consciously avoided his family and friends — even Kent.

Then one evening he found himself standing beside her in the crowded hallway after a school band concert. Amy looked up at him and without a word, took his hand and allowed him to lead her outside.

The air was fresh and cool as they stopped beside the spreading limbs of a cluster of young redbud trees. Amy gazed solemnly at the mass of trembling, heart-shaped leaves all silvery in the gathering dusk, and her eyes grew misty.

Kent searched her face, her thin, pale cheeks wet with tears, the haunting shadow of pain still apparent in her dark eyes. He put his arms around her.

"You don't have to talk," he whispered.

"I know . . . but I want to. For so long now, I've refused to talk about it. But now I have to. I still love him, Kent. I always will. But God loves him too, and what else can we do but trust that He knows what's best?

"I've prayed an awful lot in the last few months. At first I was so hurt I couldn't see beyond my own pain. I felt betrayed, by God and by Wendy, too. How could they do this to me? Then I began to remember little things he did and said."

Amy paused and took a deep breath. Kent waited patiently, allowing her to express her feelings in her own way. He stood quietly beside her, holding her hand, and listening as she continued.

"Wendy's greatest ambition was always to do whatever his Lord asked of him. If God called him, he wouldn't have hesitated for an instant. I believe that God is in control and that's why it happened the way it did."

Kent swallowed the lump in his throat and blinked away the tears in his own eyes. Amy smiled faintly and went on, "Wendy loved us, Kent. He did all that he could for us, and I'm grateful. That's what I'm going to remember—that he loved us too."

Kent couldn't speak for a long moment. He felt suddenly as if a huge weight had been lifted from his shoulders. Amy's words echoed over and over in his mind. She was right. God *was* still in control, and they could trust Him, even with Wendy's life!

Kent could feel his body actually relax. His breathing came easier and he sensed a deep warmth within himself. He realized, for the first time, that Wendy's love had led him to understand that God could provide all the comfort and security he had always looked for.

At last he spoke, "You know, Amy, all those times Wendy and I talked about trusting God, I always had to make a choice. And I always chose to follow my own will. I don't think I understood what faith was—but I'm sure learning now."

"I think we both are," Amy said. "We had a great teacher."

Time moved swiftly for Kent. Several years passed and still it seemed like only yesterday. The wounds began to heal; the pain grew less sharp, but the memories became a part of him forever!

And here he was—home again—another spring.

Kent recognized the same haunting strawberry scent floating on the air as he returned to walk along the familiar streets. The honeysuckle vines were springing to life and the old split tree near the school was starting to put on its summer finery once again. Nothing had changed; and yet, everything had changed.

Sometimes it was good to remember.

Everywhere he looked he was vividly reminded of Wendy. That old tree, the football field, a little squirrel scurrying across a limb, perhaps a descendant of the one who lived so long ago in his attic. Somehow he never had gotten around to telling his Dad.

Yes, there was much to remember.

He thought of Wendy's Mom and Dad, of Amy, and all the others. Kent knew now, better than anyone, that God had taken all of their wounded hearts and made them beautifully whole again, and more capable of loving than before.

He could still see those cold, impersonal words in a doctor's report: *"Heart failure. Congenitally defective coronary valve."* One of those rare unpredictable things there was no way of discovering, or diagnosing. Even a cardiogram in a routine athletics physical only months earlier had given no indication of a problem.

There had been many unanswered questions. Why was there no indication during their mountain climbing exertions only a few weeks earlier? Had Wendy himself suspected something was wrong? Did he have a premonition? Some things are beyond rational explanation.

How he *died* was no longer as important as how he *lived!*

Kent thought again of the many friends who had come to him to express their gratitude for Wendy. Each one felt a special closeness to him because of some small kindness or personal word he had given him. It had been much more than the normal idolizing which sometimes follows a sudden death. Those kids were sincere and honest, not about to put up false fronts as they were so quick to accuse the older generation of doing.

There was Wade, a husky athlete who had known Wendy all his life. He told Kent how he had rebelled against God for taking a friend so good and kind. Then he found he couldn't sleep at night. He kept remembering all that Wendy had represented and believed in. Finally, late one evening, he got down on his knees beside his bed and prayed for the joy and triumph that Wendy had spoken of so often, "to be alive in Christ."

Kent remembered the bright, inquisitive faces of ten small boys in their Sky Ranch T-shirts as they looked eagerly to Wendy for an answer or a word of praise; and he always gave it willingly.

There was a glistening trophy sitting in the long glass case in Skyline High School's hallway—*The Wendy Hickman Award*—an award which would be presented each year to the most outstanding member of the football team. How touched he felt standing in front of the case for the first time. He thought then of the years to come when other names would be added to the brass plate, the names of young men striving for excellence in their sport and in their lives. In the tradition for which Wendy stood so clearly, the trophy would always be a roll of honor in his memory.

Then, there was home. Kent felt warmly sentimental as he climbed the stairs to the room where they had spent so many "growing up" hours together.

There was a blue and red Raiders pennant still hanging on the wall. An old football in the corner with initials scrawled all over it. And a Smiley-face drawing, signed "Love, Wendy."

He moved to the window straining to see through a mistiness of tears. He stared out at the trees, their leaves swirling in the breeze in a fluid motion like waves lapping at the smooth green expanse of the lawn.

It was Saturday. No. He would never forget!

It was nine o'clock—He could set his watch when he looked out the upstairs window and saw him running up the drive . . . But today—today, he wouldn't be coming.

Kent turned away. Reaching into the desk drawer, he carefully drew out a letter from a small, metal box. It was crumpled and yellowed with age and from being opened and refolded so often. It brought back a new flood of memories, of picnics at the lake, bumpy, giggly rides in a pickup truck, climbing a mountain in the snow, long talks by a campfire . . .

Such real memories, he could almost hear the fire crackling. Or, was it the echo of a crowd roaring for a touchdown? He remembered that next fall when the Skyline Raiders with rugged determination had gone all-out to win the District Championship—for Wendy! And after the big game, on the bus coming home, Coach Miles' shaky voice telling them how proud he was. "We did it, boys! I'm just glad the officials didn't realize we had twelve men on the field . . . 'cause I know Wendy was there too!"

There was a solemn, but proud, ceremony when the team gathered to place the All-District Trophy in the case, to sit beside the *Wendy Hickman Award.*

Kent could still picture the bright young faces in the circle around him, each with its own mixed expression of pride and sorrow. Some of them had told him privately how they had found the same joy in Christ which was so evident in Wendy's life. All of them were thoroughly shaken, not as much by Wendy's sudden going, as by the realization it brought that every bit of life is precious and important, no matter how brief.

No. Wendy wasn't really gone. He would always be there in many ways to so many who loved him.

The familiar words in the letter he held in his hand were engraved in Kent's heart, even though they had been written so long ago. Still they brought a renewed and special feeling of love each time he read them:

> *"I have been reading in Isaiah tonight, Kent, and I came to a verse, Isaiah 49:14-15. It spells out how much the Lord really cares for us and promises that He will never forget us no matter what happens. In Isaiah 53:1-6, the scriptures tell just how much God loved us to put such a burden on His own Son to save us from eternal death.*
>
> *"Kent, my prayer is this, that all the kids and adults we know, will sometime along the way be introduced to the Lord in such a*

way that they will be truly receptive to His calling.

"I can't think of anything worse than dying without being given the chance of really knowing Christ.

"I must close now, and I hope that your week will be a glorious one indeed. I will pray for you, and I know you will do the same for me. May God bless you always!

Your friend and
brother in
Christ,
Wendy

P.S. It's Great To Be Alive in Christ!"

ALIVE IN CHRIST! Yes, Wendy is fully alive! Even on this earth, in every heart that loves him, and has learned from him, even as Kent himself finally had come to realize.

All those years he fought to do things his own way. At last he understood what Wendy tried so hard to show him—that living our lives in our own way is not really living at all.

Being truly, joyfully alive means living in Christ, and Christ living through us!

Kent's voice echoed softly in the empty room, "Thanks, Wendy."

Stepping Stone

Isn't it strange that princes and kings,
And clowns that caper in sawdust rings,
And common people, like you and me
Are builders for eternity?

Each is given a bag of tools,
A shapeless mass, a book of rules.
And each must make, ere life is flown,
A Stumbling Block, or a Stepping Stone.

— R. L. Sharpe